Specific Reading Disability

Specific Reading Disability
A View of the Spectrum

**Edited by Bruce K. Shapiro,
Pasquale J. Accardo, and
Arnold J. Capute**

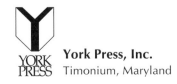

York Press, Inc.
Timonium, Maryland

This book was manufactured in the United States of America.

Typography by The Type Shoppe, Inc.

Printing and binding by McNaughton & Gunn, Inc.

Cover design by Joseph Dieter, Jr.

Book design by Sheila Stoneham.

Library of Congress Cataloging-In-Publication Data
Specific reading disability : a view of the spectrum / edited by Bruce
    K. Shapiro, Pasquale J. Accardo, and Arnold J. Capute.
        p. cm.
    Includes bibliographical references and index.
    ISBN 0-912752-45-9 (pbk.)
    1. Dyslexia--Congresses. 2. Alexia--Congresses. I. Shapiro,
Bruce K. II. Accardo, Pasquale J.   III. Capute, Arnold J, 1923-
    .
RC394.W6S64 1998
616.85'53--dc21   98-9512
                                                                  CIP

Contents

Contributors

Pasquale Accardo, M.D.
Westchester Institute for Human
Development
Cedarwood Hall
New York Medical College
Valhalla, New York 10595

Michael Bender, Ed.D.
Kennedy Krieger Institute
707 North Broadway
Baltimore, Maryland 21205

Amy M. Brower, B.S.
Boys Town National Research
Hospital
555 N. 30th Street
Omaha, Nebraska 68131

Stephen L. Buka, Sc.D.
Department of Maternal and
Child Health
Kresge Building, #309
Huntington Avenue
Boston, Massachusetts 02115

L. R. Cardon, Ph.D.
Sequana Therapeutics, Inc.
11099 North Torrey Pines Road,
Suite 160
La Jolla, California 92037

Robin P. Church, Ed.D.
Kennedy Krieger Institute
707 North Broadway
Baltimore, Maryland 21205

J. C. DeFries, Ph.D.
Institute for Behavioral Genetics
Campus Box 447
University of Colorado
Boulder, Colorado 80309-0447

John Doris, Ph.D.
Family Life Development Center
College of Human Ecology
Cornell University
Ithaca, New York 14853

Guinevere Eden, D.Phil.
Institute for Cognitive and
Computational Sciences
The Research Building WP22
3970 Reservoir Road, N.W.
Washington, DC 20007

Majorie A. Fessler, Ed.D.
Kennedy Krieger Institute
707 North Broadway
Baltimore, Maryland 21205

Doris J. Johnson, Ph.D.
Northwestern University
Frances Searle Building
2299 N. Campus Drive
Evanston, Illinois 60201

Lewis P. Lipsitt, Ph.D.
Department of Psychology
Brown University
Providence, Rhode Island 02912

Ruth D. Nass, M.D.
New York University Medical
Center
400 East 34th Street
New York, New York 10016

Judith M. Rumsey, Ph.D.
National Institute of Mental
Health
Parklawn Building, Room 18C-17
5600 Fishers Lane
Rockville, Maryland 20857

Paul Satz, Ph.D.
UCLA Neuropsychiatric Institute
and Hospital
Center for the Health Sciences
760 Westwood Plaza, C8-747
Los Angeles, California 90024-
1759

Hollis S. Scarborough, Ph.D.
Psychology Department
Brooklyn Collge of CUNY
Brooklyn, New York 11210-2889
and
Haskins Laboratories
270 Crown Street
New Haven, Connecticut 06459

Larry J. Seidman, Ph.D.
Massachusetts Mental Health
Center
74 Fernwood Road
Boston, Massachusetts 02115

Bruce K. Shapiro, M.D.
Learning Center/Family Center
Kennedy Krieger Institute
1750 East Fairmout Avenue
Baltimore, Maryland 21231-1525

Linda S. Siegel, Ph.D.
EPSE
2125 Main Mall
University of British Columbia
Vancouver, BC V6T 1Z4

Shelly D. Smith, Ph.D.
Creighton University
Boys Town National Research
Hospital
555 N. 30th Street
Omaha, Nebraska 68131

Joseph K. Torgesen, Ph.D.
Department of Psychology
Florida State University
Tallahassee, Florida 32306-
1051

Preface

Specific Reading Disability: A View of the Spectrum is a compendium of papers presented March 18–20, 1996 at the eighteenth annual Spectrum of Developmental Disabilities course. As specific reading disability approached forty and its corollary, dyslexia, approached its centennial, we thought it appropriate to apply current research findings to the assumptions underlying identification, diagnosis, management, and prognosis of specific reading disability. The papers contained within this volume range widely and identify many different spectra.

One such spectrum concerns the nature of specific reading disability. Some view it narrowly as the inability to attach sounds to symbols with resultant slowness in decoding and impaired comprehension. Another view is that specific reading disability falls within the spectrum of central communicative disorders. Others have posited that specific reading disability is merely the tail end of the normal curve of reading abilities, while some doubt its existence.

Another spectrum spans the issues of identification and diagnosis. How to identify specific reading disability and distinguish it from other causes of academic dysfunction remains a challenge. The most common method, use of the discrepancy between potential and achievement, is neither sensitive nor specific. The effects of age, influence of co-morbid conditions, and consequences of therapy on identification and diagnosis are within this spectrum.

The chapters in this volume identify another spectrum: the spectrum from classroom to policy to research. This spectrum is not linear. Important contributions have been made by the disciplines of education, psychology, speech and language pathology, social work, pediatrics, neurology, genetics, and psychiatry.

Research techniques that extend our knowledge of brain functions are part of this volume. Quantitative and functional neuroimaging, processing, pharmacology, and animal studies of learning are but some of the techniques being used to understand specific reading disability. Genetics and epidemiology also promise to increase our knowledge of specific reading disability. The new techniques hold out the promise of identifying specific reading disability before academic failure and the concomitant poor self esteem are evident.

Specific reading disability is a series of spectra. We have not yet reached our goal of eliminating specific reading disability. Better data about outcomes will be required to determine how well we are doing. However, knowledge is accumulating, the scope of the problem is becoming clearer, and approaches are being applied. Specific reading disability is in a dynamic state.

—Bruce K. Shapiro, MD
—Pasquale J. Accardo, MD
—Arnold J. Capute, MD, MPH

Section • 1

Reading Disability Within a Context

Chapter • 1

Dyslexia *The Evolution of a Concept*

John L. Doris

If we look back at the concept of developmental dyslexia as it was presented in the literature at the beginning of this century, it had a clarity and validity that I hope to demonstrate by citations from that literature. Somehow, by the middle of the century, the concept of dyslexia had become amalgamated with and subsumed under a larger category of developmental problems called at first *minimal brain dysfunction* and subsequently *learning disabilities*. The clarity and validity were compromised.

Nevertheless, it may be argued that this amalgamation had many positive aspects from the point of view of those concerned with the various handicaps of the school-age child. Certainly, the large numbers of children—however disparate the developmental problems, subsumed under the label of learning disabilities—permitted a mobilization of parental, professional, and public concern resulting in legislative action in the 1970s and a funding stream that promoted research, demonstration projects, the training of professionals, and the development of remedial programs for various handicaps. This forms an effective demonstration of the power of numbers when we seek to effect public policy to remedy a problem of health or education.

On the other hand, forming a conglomerate called learning disabilities out of such disparate disorders as dyslexia, hyperactivity, attention deficits, and other assorted cognitive and perceptual impairments undoubtedly created obstacles for the rational pursuit of research on diagnostic, etiological, preventive, and therapeutic factors for the individual clinical entities so subsumed—obstacles that, despite persistent attack over the past ten to fifteen years, have not yet been satisfactorily overcome.

THE DYSLEXIC CHILD

It is now 100 years since the first published case of developmental dyslexia appeared in the medical literature. W. Pringle Morgan, a school physician having read Hinshelwood's (1895) paper on acquired word blindness in a British medical journal, was inspired to submit to the same journal a paradoxical case report on a 14-year-old school boy competent in arithmetic, considered bright by his teacher and intelligent in conversation, who yet was incapable of learning to read, despite the lack of any history of neurological illness or insult that might have explained the condition. Reporting on his examination of the child, W. Pringle Morgan (1896) indicated that when the boy was asked to read out of an easy children's book:

> The result was curious. He did not read a single word correctly, with the exception of "and," "the," "of," "that," etc.; the other words seemed to be quite unknown to him, and he could not even make an attempt to pronounce them.
> I next tried his ability to read figures, and found he could do so easily. . . . He multiplied 749 by 876 quickly and easily. He says that he is fond of arithmetic and has no difficulty with it, but that printed or written words "have no meaning for him," and my examination of him quite convinces me that he is correct in that opinion. Words written or printed seem to convey no impression to his mind, and it is only after laboriously spelling them that he is able by dint of the sound of the letters, to discover their import. . . . I may add that the boy is bright and of average intelligence in conversation. . . . The schoolmaster who has taught him for some years says that he would be the smartest lad in the school if the instruction were entirely oral. (p. 1378)

Morgan concluded that the boy's condition was "evidently congenital and due most probably to defective development of that region of the brain, disease of which in adults produces practically the same symptoms, that is, the left angular gyrus."

In short order, similar case reports appeared in medical, psychological, and educational literature and in 1917 Hinshelwood, an ophthalmologist, published a monograph presenting diagnostic considerations, a theoretical explanation, and a remedial approach. Hinshelwood believed the term *congenital word-blindness* should be reserved only for the severest form of reading handicap in the child who, otherwise intellectually competent, could not be taught by ordinary school methods. He believed its incidence to be rare and of an order of less than one in a thousand. He noted its greater frequency in males and its familial tendency. Struck by the fact that congenital word-blindness never was accompanied by homonymous hemianopsia—as was frequently the case with acquired alexia—he doubted that birth injury or disease was a factor in any but a small proportion of the cases. Rather, he opted for a developmental defect that in some cases was of an obvious hereditary nature. By analogy with acquired alexia in adults, he postulated defective development in the region of the angular gyrus of the dominant hemisphere. The difficulty in learning to read was manifestly "that of storing up and retaining the visual memories of words and letters. In the examination of these children this deficiency becomes most evident in the contrast afforded between their visual memories for words and letters, and their auditory memory for the same, which . . . is preserved intact" (p. 86). A marked difference in the ability to read words and numbers was considered diagnostic, for most of the children were competent and some even excellent in arithmetic.

In the remediation of word-blindness, Hinshelwood recommended strengthening the visual word center by the old alphabetic method of teaching reading reinforced by the auditory memory and by the kinesthetic memory of movement in speech and writing; for, he asserted, all the separate language centers identified by the neurologists of the 19th century were interconnected and could be used to reinforce each other in the process of reading. But for Hinshelwood, most crucial in the teaching of such children was individual instruction, where the child would not be discouraged by comparison with his or her classmates, and the teaching could be easily adapted to the child's difficulties.

Despite the many important and far-seeing contributions of Hinshelwood, his estimate of an incidence of less than one in a thousand did little to focus the attention of educators or the public at large on the plight of these school children.

Indeed, educational literature of the first two decades of the twentieth century, when it did on occasion take note of the so-called word-blind child, also assumed that he was extremely rare. Clara Schmitt, an examiner of problem children in the Chicago public schools, noted in 1918 that only 13 word-blind children had been identified in a school population of approximately 43,000. Nevertheless, this educational literature, sparse as it is, contains many excellent clinical descriptions of the children and innovative approaches to their remediation.

One of Clara Schmitt's cases, a ten-year-old fourth grader, presented a rather classical picture. Successful in arithmetic, a competent music student, and considered very intelligent by her teachers, she could recognize but few words in her reading and was never very certain of even the simplest ones. Given special training in phonics by the speech teacher, she made satisfactory progress. But even in the seventh grade there was continued evidence of difficulty and she gave the interesting introspective report that after being out of school for a week and not reading she would forget how to read and then would have to begin all over again to work out the words phonically. "I look at the letters and then keep wondering and wondering what is the sound, and finally it comes back to me" (p. 692).

Another striking feature of this early educational literature is that in discussions of the learning problems met with in the special education classes of that period, distinction is made not only between different types of learning handicaps but sub-types within the category of the reading handicapped.

Thus in 1914, Elizabeth Walsh, who headed the special education program in the New York City schools, describes the screening process for placement as follows:

> The emphasis is placed on those border-line cases which are being reported more and more by the schools; of those children who deviate only slightly from the normal, the child who can grasp arithmetic but who cannot learn to read, and vice versa, the child who is strongly ear-minded or motor-minded and who has fallen behind because the instruction given in most schools is based on the fact that the majority of the children are eye-minded. (p. 60)

In a similar vein, Barbara Morgan's 1914 book on clinical testing and treatment of children with learning problems in the New York City schools distinguishes the eye-minded from the ear-minded child, the child who perceives analytically from the child who perceives synthetically and recommends that training be adapted to these individual differences. As examples, she describes two children with marked discrepancies between their general level of competency and their ability to learn even the alphabet, let alone read. With one "ear-minded" eleven-year-old girl, success was achieved by printing the letters on the keys of a piano and teaching the child to pick out tunes with one finger as she called out the letters (pp. 34–36.) For a ten-year-old boy "muscular associations" were used to strengthen "mental associations" and the alphabet was taught in association with simple dance steps, followed by the printing of the letters with each individual stroke of the pen accompanied by repeated verbalizations of that letter's name (pp. 217–20).

This evidence from the educational literature of the first two decades of our century suggests that a number of special education teachers of that period were acquainted with a variety of learning problems later classified as learning disabilities, and that for purposes of remediation they saw the need to form sub-categories not only of the group as a whole but also of the reading disabilities themselves. Here in embryonic form was a recognition of the need for sub-typing that is a present-day focus of research and practice. Still, these educators, like the physicians of that period, imagined the so-called word blind or dyslexic child to be extremely rare.

In fact, many leaders of remedial reading programs developed in the public schools during this period drew attention away from the unique difficulties that these children faced in learning to read. Gates (1935), an outstanding leader in the field, challenged the very utility of the concept of word-blindness in considering the reading disabilities of children. Discussing the term *nonreaders*, a term covering the more severe disabilities of reading, such as word-blindness or dyslexia, he would point out that nonreaders were not a distinct group, but merely the extreme cases of disability on a distribution from the most handicapped reader to the most competent. The differences that placed a child on different points of the distribution were of degree not kind. Such a theoretical stance made for a close alliance between the growing field of remedial reading, with its special techniques of diagnosis and instruction, and the developmental reading programs as practiced in schools. A presumed low incidence rate for dyslexic children along with the amalgamation of such children into the wider class of poor readers in public schools served to blur the focus on the unique problems of these children.

In the mid-twenties, however, the work of Samuel Orton was to prove a powerful force in refocusing attention on the special and qualitatively different disabilities of these children. In 1925, Orton, director of a state psychopathic hospital, had responded to a request of the Iowa Conference of Social Work by sending a visiting mental health clinic to rural Greene County. In the two weeks of its existence the clinic evaluated 173 referrals from all sources. Of note is the fact that the bulk of the referrals were from the county schools. Eighty-four of the children were described by their teachers as "dull, backward or retarded" and 30 were described as "nervous, peculiar, or unruly" (Lyday 1926).

Among these referrals were 15 children, with IQs ranging from 70 to 122, that the clinic identified as having a special difficulty in learning to read. Although Orton granted that only two of his cases fit Hinshelwood's strict criteria for "congenital word blindness," he was struck by similarities in the reading behavior of all the cases that had been identified as having a special reading problem in the Greene County schools. These similarities included such notable characteristics as the reversal of individual letters and the tendency to read letter groups or palindromic words, such as *god* and *dog* or *was* and *saw* from right to left (Orton 1925).

Given this group of cases, varying in the severity of defect but similar in their behavioral symptoms, Orton was convinced that the category of word-blindness should be broadened to include a graded series of reading handicaps from severe cases, as studied by Hinshelwood, to those cases that could, in fact, achieve a fair degree of facility in reading.

In addition to broadening the category, Orton rejected Hinshelwood's theory of defective embryonic development of the cerebral area subserving visual memory of words and letters. Instead, based in part on the observed letter reversals and the sinistrad reading of groups of letters and words, he offered an explanation for the reading disabilities in the developmental failure to establish unilateral cortical dominance and suggested the term *strephosymbolia* as more aptly describing the entity.

On the basis of continued research on reading handicaps in Iowa school children, Orton was to assert that "children suffering from this condition in a degree sufficiently severe to be a really significant obstacle to school progress formed at least two per cent of the total school population in every community visited . . . " (Orton 1928).

This two percent estimate is a marked increase over the prevalence rate of less than one in a thousand offered by Hinshelwood. If Orton's estimate were to be accepted as an accurate estimate of children with distinct handicaps in reading, the schools would be faced with a sizable problem of needed special provisions. In addition, Orton, early in his research program, became aware of the not infrequent occurrence of stuttering in children with marked reading disability and speculated that this speech difficulty was also related to a fundamental problem in the establishment of cerebral dominance. By the time of his 1937 publication, *Reading, Writing and Speech Problems in Children*, Orton considered a broader range of developmental disorders including (a) developmental alexia or strephosymbolia, (b) developmental agraphia or marked difficulty in learning to write, (c) developmental word deafness in which auditory acuity is normal, but there is a specific impairment of verbal understanding, (d) developmental motor aphasia or motor speech delay, (e) developmental apraxia or abnormal clumsiness, and (f) stuttering.

What is interesting from the point of view of our present day use of the term learning disabilities, is that this was an early attempt to classify, within the same conceptual and etiological framework, a range of language and motor disabilities in addition to the commonly encountered reading handicap.

THE CONCEPT OF MINIMAL BRAIN DAMAGE

In addition to Orton's contribution, a second development in the medical field during the 1920s was to affect the categorization of children with learning problems and to add to the prevalence rates. This was the introduction of the concept of minimal brain damage.

The epidemic of encephalitis following the First World War played a particularly important role in the formation of the concept of minimal brain damage. Early in the 1920s a number of medical reports indicated that children recovering from encephalitis exhibited various sequelae—physical, intellectual, and behavioral defects occurring in all degrees from the most severe to the scarcely identifiable (Happ and Mason 1921; Patterson and Spence 1921). These sequelae, following upon a known infection of brain tissue, provided a model of brain injury accompanied by a variety of behavioral and intellectual disturbances with or without the coexistence of gross neurological signs. In short order, the model was extended to include the assumption that, when a patient presents with sequelae of epidemic encephalitis without evidence of prior acute illness, he or she must have suffered from brain disease.

Thus, in Lauretta Bender's report (1942) on the experience of her group with the evaluation and treatment of postencephalitic children, emphasis is on hyperkinesis and other impulse disturbances and on the presence of distinctive psychometric patterns. In summary, she would state:

> The diagnostic criteria for encephalopathic behavior disorders are now considerable. Even without a history of the specific etiological factor or evidence of the specific pathology, the diagnostic methods which may be applied to fields of behavior are sufficient to establish a diagnosis. (pp. 379–80)

Reports by various clinicians and researchers on the relationship of prenatal and paranatal factors affecting subsequent development of the child also served to strengthen the hypothesis of a relationship between undetectable neurological lesions and behavioral and intellectual impairment.

Here we might mention the developmental diagnostic studies of infants as reported by Arnold Gesell and Catherine Amatruda (1941) and the empirical studies of Knobloch and Pasamanick (1959) on the development of children whose case histories revealed perinatal or paranatal stress.

THE BEHAVIORAL DIAGNOSIS OF BRAIN INJURY

The application of this concept of minimal brain damage to the learning problems of the school-age child was greatly fostered by the research and remedial training programs of Alfred A. Strauss and his colleagues.

Within the general category of mental retardation, Strauss distinguished the brain-injured or "exogenous" child and the "endogenous" child whose mental subnormality was familial or unrelated to injury to the central nervous system. Based on his clinical work and an impressive program of research carried out with Heinz Werner, he concluded that the brain-injured child was characterized by disturbances in perception, thinking, and emotional behavior that differentiated him from the endogenous or familial retardate.

Among the various criteria Strauss listed for the diagnosis of minor brain injury, the following, which appeared in the 1947 publication of Strauss and Lehtinen, was most influential in determining the scope of the nascent area of learning disabilities:

> When no mental retardation exists, the presence of psychological disturbances can be discovered by the use of some of our qualitative tests for perceptual and conceptual disturbances. Although the . . . (other) criteria may be negative, whereas the behavior of the child in question resembles that characteristic for brain injury, and even though the performances of the child on our tests are not strongly indicative of brain injury, it may still be reasonable to consider a diagnosis of brain injury. (p. 112)

This criterion indicates the great importance Strauss and his co-workers assigned to behavioral patterns and test performance; these could be diagnostic even in the absence of mental retardation.

By 1964, professional, parental, and public interest in the concept of minimal brain damaged children with its associated educational and behavioral handicaps had grown to a point that the National Easter Seal Society for Crippled Children and Adults in conjunction with the Department of Health, Education and Welfare recommended the establishment of three task forces to study the issue. In the 1966 report of the task force on Terminology and Identification, tribute was paid to the classic study of Strauss and Lehtinen. It was noted that "few single volumes have been so influential in the production of fresh considerations in the areas of pathology, diagnosis, education, and investigation of children with learning and behavioral difficulties" (p. 5).

This report endorsed a change in terminology from "minimal brain damage" to "minimal brain dysfunction syndrome," to refer "to children of near average, average, or above average general intelligence with certain learning or behavioral disabilities ranging from mild to severe, which are associated with deviations of function of the central nervous system. These deviations may manifest themselves by various combinations of impairment in perception, conceptualization, language, memory, and control of attention, impulse or motor function" (pp. 9–10). In an extensive listing of the various syndromes manifesting minimal brain dysfunction, the clinical entities of hyperactivity and primary reading retardation, or what we may prefer to call dyslexia, were singled out. The report indicates that these various disorders "may arise from genetic variations, biochemical irregularities, perinatal brain insults or other illnesses or injuries sustained during the years which are critical for the development and maturation of the central nervous system, or from unknown causes." What is interesting in this etiological statement is that it moves beyond brain injury to postulate a variety of causes some of which are known, some suspected, and some unknown.

FROM BIRTH INJURY TO LEARNING DISABILITY

This concept of minimal brain damage or minimal brain dysfunction as publicized by Strauss and his collaborators was to have a heavy impact on the theoretical formulations and practice recommendations of many who were to define and develop the field of learning disabilities in the following decades—especially, those who were to emphasize the perceptual-motor and psycholinguistic processes underlying the acquisition of reading skills.

In many respects, particularly the reduction of environmental stimulation within the learning environment, Cruickshank (1977) was the closest adherent to the Strauss-Lehtinen tradition. Taking a position congenial to many a practice-oriented educator he argued:

> While proper diagnosis is important, the symptomology—the characteristics of the child—is more important, because it is the latter with which educators, psychologists, and others who are involved in habilitative programs and therapy must deal. (p. 5)

This position of Cruickshank's, that the etiology was less important than the behavioral handicap, was advocated even more strongly by Samuel Kirk. In a 1962 article with Barbara Bateman, it was argued that, generally, remediation was determined by the behavioral symptoms, not by the neurological findings.

> Our interest is in the kind and extent of diagnosis of learning problems, that lead directly to a formulation of what should be done about the disability. (p. 73)

In that same article appeared a definition of learning disability that was to become the progenitor of a number of definitions widely prevalent in succeeding decades:

> A *learning disability* refers to a retardation, disorder, or delayed development in one or more of the processes of speech, language, reading, writing, arithmetic, or other school subjects resulting from a psychological handicap caused by possible cerebral dysfunction and/or emotional or behavioral disturbances. It is not the result of mental retardation, sensory deprivation, or cultural or instructional factors. (p. 73)

Subsequently, at the 1963 organizational meeting of the Association for Children with Learning Disabilities, Kirk (1975) was to contrast etiological terms such as *minimal brain damage* or *cerebral dysfunction* with behaviorally descriptive terms such as *hyperkinetic behavior* or *perceptual disorders* in the classification of such children. Warning of the dangers inherent in all labels, but assuming that the purpose of the organization was "not to conduct research on behavior and the brain, but to find effective methods of diagnosis, management, and training of the children," he offered the term *learning disability* as a general designation for the wide range of handicaps. Adopted in the title of this advocacy organization, the term learning disability soon became the prevailing designation.

The "functional diagnosis" of minimal brain damage or learning disability by means of behavioral indices and by performance on various psychological and educational tests, particularly the newer perceptual motor and psycholinguistic tests specifically designed for diagnostic purposes, greatly facilitated the identification of a growing number of educationally handicapped children. The use of these efficient diagnostic tests coupled with remedial exercises devised by Strauss, Cruickshank, Kirk, and their followers apparently filled a great need for frustrated educators struggling with the learning difficulties of their pupils. Critical evaluations of these instruments and remedial exercises later diminished much of their popularity (Hammill 1972; Kavale and Mattson 1983; Larsen, Parker, and Hammill 1982); but the decades of the seventies and eighties saw a phenomenal growth in the field of learning disabilities.

Certainly, not the least factor in this growth was the passage of the Education of the Handicapped Act (P.L. 91–230), which authorized programs of research, training, and model centers addressed to the needs of "children with specific learning disabilities." In the school year of 1968/69, just prior to the passage of this Act, some 120,000 children were enrolled in special education services under this categorical label (Martin 1970). In 1976/77, the school year following passage of the Education for all Handicapped Children (P.L. 94–142), which made further provisions for the education of the learning disabled, 796,000 learning disabled children received special educational services. By the school year 1987/88 the number had reached 1,928,000—accounting for 4.8% of the public school enrollment from kindergarten through 12th grade (U.S. Department of Education 1989).

Concurrent with this growth in learning disabilities, there has been a marked drop in the number of children served in the category of the mentally retarded. It is generally conceded that many of the mildly retarded are now served as learning disabled. It might be ventured that children with other school problems have also been drawn into the vortex.

DEFINITIONAL ISSUES IN LEARNING DISABILITIES

In 1976 Freeman had vigorously expressed himself on these long-standing definitional issues:

> There is only one phrase for the state of the art and practice in the field of minimal brain dysfunction (MBD), hyperactivity (HA), and learning disability (LD) in children: a mess. There is no more polite term which would be realistic. The area is characterized by rarely challenged myths, ill-defined boundaries, and a strangely seductive attractiveness. These categories and their management, because of massive support from frustrated parents, professionals, government, and the drug and remedial-education industries, constitute an epidemic of alarming proportions—but is the problem the disease or its treatment?" (p. 5)

To Freeman, there was, in fact, no epidemic in the field of minimal brain dysfunction, learning disorders, and hyperactivity in children "but rather, an unfortunate episode in the history of progressive medicalization of deviant or troublesome behavior" (p. 22). He further maintained that:

> Surely part of the confusion in the field is due to a lack of useful criteria to delimit these nonsynonymous groups of children: MBD, LD, and HA. "One or more" of an endless series of equivocal and often subjective characteristics is not very helpful but can open the possibility that almost any child can be labeled. (p. 10)

In spite of his vigorous attack on categorical labels, equivocally defined, with presumptive etiologies and questionable therapies, it is interesting that Freeman still assumed the existence of a core subgroup of "severely and persistently impaired children." The threat of labels indiscriminately applied to ever increasing numbers of children was that they obscured, "the very important distinction between the relatively small number of children with biologically based difficulties and the larger number who are failing to meet the expectations of their families or the school system for other reasons" (p. 22).

The indiscriminate application of the label of learning disabilities had been previously documented for the federally funded Child Service Demonstration Centers. These model centers were funded under the Education of the Handicapped Act (P.L. 91–230) with its specified definition of learning disabilities, and one might have supposed that their selection of children to be serviced would, for the most part, reflect the influence of that federal definition. Yet Kirk and Elkins (1975) reporting on the characteristics of over 3,000 children enrolled in these Centers stated that:

> It would appear from the data that the majority of children in the projects, although underachieving to some degree, would not qualify as specific learning disabled children, since (a) many of the children were retarded equally in reading, spelling, and arithmetic and were, therefore, not specific but general in academic retardation, and (b) a substantial proportion were minor or moderate in their degree of under achievement. (p. 636)
>
> Previously, many of these children would have been classified as slow learners or as mentally retarded. . . . . . Admittedly, these children—slow learners, disadvantaged children and others—need attention from compensatory programs . . . but one can raise the question of whether these children require the same kind of emphasis as children with specific learning disabilities. . . . (p. 636–637)

A subsequent analysis of the reports from the Child Service Demonstration Centers, which had been funded from 1971 to 1980, though admittedly based on less than satisfactory data, led Mann and his associates (1983) to similar, if less temperate, conclusions:

> Let us then accept the facts as we find them. And they suggest that we adopt learning disabilities as a generic term for all "mildly" handicapped as the label to replace other stigmatizing ones. To clarify the term for labeling purposes we can go the DSM III route—a vague enough one to suit all purposes and meeting the requirements of an age which does not prize diagnostic excellence. We can have: learning disabilities with cultural deprivation, learning disabilities with behavior disorders, learning disabilities with neurological problems, etc. Markers, then, of various sorts can be used to define these LD groups for scientific study as Barbara Keogh has suggested. (Keogh 1978). Thus, we have LD with variables I, X, Y for this study, LD with variables M, W, Y for that study. (p. 17)

Though these studies of data gathered from the Child Service Demonstration Centers had the advantage of sampling the practices of a large number of states, they had the limitation of methodological weakness recognized by their authors. Shepard and her colleagues, focusing on the State of Colorado, gave a more solidly based assessment of practice in the field of learning disabilities in that setting.

In one component of their work, a probability sample of 790 cases was selected from all the learning disabled children served in the State of Colorado and their case records were analyzed for defining characteristics. Approximately 43% of the sample had characteristics associated in Federal law and professional literature with definitions of learning disabilities. Approximately another 40% consisted of other handicaps and learning problems. The remaining 17% were misidentified for various reasons such as poor assessment (Shepard, Smith, and Vojir 1983).

> The implication of these results for basic research on learning disabilities is that the label applied for the purpose of providing services cannot be assumed valid. If the label is taken as a dependable sign of the disability; then research on LD heritability patterns, prevalence rates, and the effectiveness of interventions will be confounded. The meaning or meanings of learning disabilities will remain elusive. (p. 328)

In a series of articles Shepard addressed the educational and scientific costs of such rampant misdiagnoses. Inflating the numbers of learning disabled children reduces the available educational resources needed for the more seriously handicapped children. For example, at the time of Shepard's work in the early 1980s, it cost only $5 to place a child in a Title I program that might adequately and appropriately provide for his or her educational needs. The costs of LD identification with its due process procedures now might run from $600 to $1000 per child (Shepard 1983; Shepard and Smith 1983).

The indiscriminate use of the label of learning disabilities, as documented in these studies by Kirk, Mann, Shepard, and their colleagues, contributed to the on-going debate in the literature on the distinctness of the LD category in relationship to other special education categories. In fact, it is apparent that ever since Kirk first advanced the term *learning disabilities* in the early sixties, the field has repeatedly struggled to improve its conceptual and operational definitions.

In an article optimistically entitled "On Defining Learning Disabilities: An Emerging Consensus," Donald Hammill (1990) has identified eleven different conceptual definitions that are prominent today or have experienced a degree of popularity in the past. Within these definitions he has identified nine important conceptual elements on which the definitions could differ. These include such components as the etiology, the role of psychological processes, and the specification of academic spoken language, and/or non-language skill deficits.

Calculating the percentage agreement on these components among the definitions, he concludes that contrary to popular opinion, considerable agreement exists among the definitions. This is particularly true of every important definition of learning disabilities currently enjoying any degree of popularity. Of all eleven definitions considered, four that have been developed since 1977 are, in Hammill's view, the only professionally viable alternatives. These definitions are those offered by the United States Office of Education (USOE), the National Joint Committee on Learning Disabilities (NJCLD), the Learning Disabilities Association of America (LDA), and the Interagency Committee on Learning Disabilities (ICLD). The remaining definitions are considered to have only historical importance.

Of the viable alternatives, Hammill gives special consideration to two, those of the Office of Education and the National Joint Committee on Learning Disabilities. That of the Office of Education (1977) is based squarely upon the definition as it appears in Federal legislation:

> "Specific learning disability" means a disorder in one or more of the basic psychological processes involved in understanding or in using language, spoken or written, which may manifest itself in an imperfect ability to listen, speak, read, write, spell, or to do mathematical calculations. The term includes such conditions as perceptual handicaps, brain injury, minimal brain dysfunction, dyslexia, and developmental aphasia. The term does not include children who have learning problems which are primarily the result of visual, hearing, or motor handicaps, of mental retardation, of emotional disturbance, or of environmental, cultural, or economic disadvantage. (p. 65083)

The definition of the National Joint Committee is in agreement with the USOE definition on seven of the nine elements examined by Hammill. It deletes the controversial phrase *basic psychological processes*, and it specifies conceptual problems (i.e., problems in reasoning or thinking) in addition to the academic and spoken language problems listed in the USOE definition.

Of these two definitions, Hammill considers the NJCLD the better (Hammill et al. 1987/1981). The inclusion of the *psychological process clause* is the main limitation of the USOE definition. The term lacks specificity and was not operationalized in the identification criteria that accompanied the USOE's publication of the definition. The term also carries the burden of its association with the once popular diagnostic and remedial perceptual-motor techniques advocated during the 1960s.

Although an advocate of the NJCLD definition and believing that it has the better chance of becoming the consensus definition, Hammill (1990) concludes that:

> Political realities are such that the NJCLD definition may never replace the 1977 USOE definition in law. But this may not be important. What is important, however, is that professionals and parents unite around one definition so that we can say with assurance, "This is what we mean when we say *learning disabilities.*" (p. 83)

In that statement, Hammill alludes to one of the vital functions carried by the name and definition of any clinical entity: to serve as the banner around which we rally as we attempt to arouse public interest and influence public policy. And certainly the term learning disabilities has served that purpose well. Its broad and loosely defined boundaries have permitted us to enlist large numbers of parents and educators as well as representatives from a wide range of science and health disciplines in a common effort to improve the lives of those school children and adults to whom that label is applied. The passage of Federal legislation in the 1970s and 1980s with funding for research, demonstration projects, and professional training attests to the success of that common effort.

But a problem remains. Is a broad and loosely defined category of developmental disorders conducive to progress in understanding and remediating the distinct disorders that it contains? I think the literature of the last ten to fifteen years with its increasing focus on the problem of identifying subgroups within the category of learning disabilities gives clear evidence that professionals in the field have concluded that such is not the case either for purposes of research or for the purpose of designing rational and valid interventions.

That literature also indicates that pulling apart this conglomerate of learning disabilities is no easy task with many competing typologies arrived at by various clinical-inferential and empirically based methodologies.

Linda Siegel and Jamie Metsala (1992) have addressed the difficult definitional, measurement, and statistical issues involved in subtyping the category of learning disabilities and have been sanguine enough to state that:

> Conceptualizing learning disability subtypes as being based on differences in achievement profiles seems to be the most meaningful approach. There appear to be at least three subtypes: reading disabled, arithmetic disabled, attentional deficit. (p. 56)

If we should arrive at such a typology that is generally acceptable, much will have been gained. However as Riccio, Gonzalex, and

Hynd (1994) recently pointed out, the difficulties in teasing apart attention-deficit hyperactivity disorders from learning disabilities is not yet an accomplished fact:

> The importance of providing validated criteria for diagnosis and learning disabilities cannot be overstated. Methodological problems and inconsistent diagnoses, as well as prevalent co–morbidity of attentional deficits/hyperactivity with learning disabilities make it difficult to interpret and replicate research with these populations. Further, conflicting findings due to variances in samples, heterogeneity of the samples, and differing diagnostic methods cloud and impede the advances in intervention-centered assessment. In this regard, better and more consistent classification/diagnostic strategies need to be developed. (p. 317)

Finally, there is the issue of subtyping the reading disability group itself. The assumption that such types exist goes all the way back to the first decades of the century when the special education teachers distinguished the visual-minded child from the auditory-minded child, the child who perceived analytically from the child who perceived synthetically. A strong strain of interest in the identification of subtypes within the category of reading disabilities has been evident in the literature ever since the 1970s but as Siegel and Metsala (1992) state in their summary of this literature:

> It appears that the study of subtypes has been plagued by serious definitional issues and that there does not appear to be any evidence of reliable subtypes within the reading disabled population. (p. 51)

Despite this somewhat discouraging assessment, one cannot fail to be impressed by the increased conceptual sophistication and the methodological and statistical advances in the behavioral studies of subtyping as revealed in the literature of this past decade. To this, one may add the rapid development of our understanding of the biological underpinnings of reading disabilities promoted by recent advances in both the fields of neurology and genetics. (Lyon et al. 1993; Duane and Gray 1991). It is not unreasonable to expect that such combined efforts will soon lead to a clarification of the subtypes of reading disabilities, including the severe form of disability that we term *dyslexia*.

REFERENCES

Bender, L. 1942. Post-encephalitic behavior disorders in childhood. In *Encephalitis*, ed. J. B. Neal. New York: Grune & Stratton.

Clements, Samuel D. 1966. *Minimal Brain Dysfunction in Children*, (NIDB Monograph No. 3), Public Health Service Publication (No. 1415). Washington, DC: United States Department of Health, Education and Welfare.

Cruickshank, W. M. 1977. *Learning Disabilities in Home, School and Community*. Syracuse: Syracuse University Press.

Duane, D., and Gray, D. (eds.) 1991. *The Reading Brain: The Biological Basis of Dyslexia.* Parkton, MD: York Press.

Freeman, R. D. 1976. Minimal brain dysfunction, hyperactivity, and learning disorders: Epidemic or episode? *School Review*, 85:5–30.

Gates, A. 1935. *The Improvement of Reading* (rev. ed.). New York: Macmillan.

Gesell, A., and Amatruda, C. S. 1941. *Developmental Diagnosis.* New York: Hoeber.

Hammill, D. 1972. Training visual perceptual processes. *Journal of Learning Disabilities* 5:552–59.

Hammill, D. D. 1990. On defining learning disabilities: An emerging consensus. *Journal of Learning Disabilities* 23:74–84.

Hammill, D. D., Leigh, J. E., McNutt, G., and Larsen, S. C. 1987/1981. A new definition of learning disabilities. *Journal of Learning Disabilities* 20:109–12.

Happ, W. M., and Mason, V. R. 1921. Epidemic encephalitis: A clinical study. *Bulletin of The Johns Hopkins Hospital* 32:137–59.

Hinshelwood, J. 1895. Word-blindness and visual memory. Lancet 2:1564–70.

Hinshelwood, J. 1917. *Congenital Word-blindness.* Chicago: Medical Book Co.

Kavale, K., and Mattson, P. D. 1983. "One jumped off the balance beam": Meta-analysis of perceptual-motor training. *Journal of Learning Disabilities* 16:165–73.

Keogh, B. K., Major, S., Reid, H. P., Gandara, P., and Omori, H. 1978. Marker variables. *Learning Disability Quarterly* 1:5–11.

Kirk, S.A. 1962. *Educating Exceptional Children.* Boston: Houghton Mifflin.

Kirk, S. A. 1975. Behavioral diagnosis and remediation of learning disorders. In *Learning Disabilities: Selected ACLD Papers*, eds. S. A. Kirk and J. McRae McCarthy. Boston: Houghton Mifflin.

Kirk, S. A., and Bateman, B. 1962/63. Diagnosis and remediation of learning disabilities. *Exceptional Children* 29:73–78.

Kirk, S. A., and Elkins, J. 1975. Characteristics of children enrolled in the child service demonstration centers. *Journal of Learning Disabilities* 8:630–37.

Knobloch, H., and Pasamanick, B. 1959. Syndrome of minimal cerebral damage in infancy. *Journal of the American Medical Association* 170:1384–87.

Larsen, S. C., Parker, R. M., and Hammill, D. D. 1982. Effectiveness of psycholinguistic training: A response to Kavale. *Exceptional Children* 49:60–66.

Lyday, J. F. 1926. The Greene County Mental Clinic. *Mental Hygiene* 10:759–86.

Lyon, G., Gray, D., Kavanagh, J., and Krasnegor, N. 1993. *Better Understanding Learning Disabilities.* Baltimore, MD: Brookes.

Mann, L., Davis, C. H., Boyer, C. W., Metz, C. M., and Wolford, B. 1983. LD or not LD, that was the question. *Journal of Learning Disabilities* 16:14–17.

Martin, E. W. 1970. Programs of The Bureau of Education for the Handicapped: U. S. Office of Education. *Programs for the Handicapped.* Washington, DC: U. S. Department of Health, Education, and Welfare.

Morgan, B. S. 1914. *The Backward Child.* NY: G. P. Putnam's Sons.

Morgan, W. P. 1896. A case of congenital word blindness. *British Medical Journal* 2:1378.

National Joint Committee on Learning Disabilities. 1987/1981. Learning disabilities: Issues on definition. *Journal of Learning Disabilities* 20:107–8.

Orton, S. T. 1925. "Word-blindness" in school children. *Archives of Neurology and Psychiatry* 14:581–615.

Orton, S. T. 1928. Specific reading disability—Strephosymbolia. *Journal of the American Medical Association* 90:1095–99.

Orton, S. T. 1937. *Reading, Writing and Speech Problems in Children.* New York: W. W. Norton.

Patterson, D., and Spence, J. C. 1921. The after effects of epidemic encephalitis in children. *Lancet* 2:491–93.

Riccio, C. A., Gonzalex, J. J., and Hynd, G. W. 1994. Attention-deficit hyperactivity disorder (ADHD) and learning disabilities. *Learning Disability Quarterly* 17:311–22.

Schmitt, C. 1917/1918. Developmental alexia: Congenital word-blindness, or inability to learn to read. *The Elementary School Journal* 18:680–700, 757–69.

Shepard, L. 1983. The role of measurement in educational policy: lessons from the identification of learning disabilities. *Educational Measurement: Issues and Practice* 2:4–8.

Shepard, L., and Smith, M. 1983. An evaluation of the identification of learning disabled students in Colorado. *Learning Disability Quarterly* 6:115–27.

Shepard, L. A., Smith, M. L., and Vojir, C. P. 1983. Characteristics of pupils identified as learning disabled. *American Educational Research Journal* 20:309–31.

Siegel, L., and Metsala, J. 1992. An alternative to the food processor approach to subtypes of learning disabilities. In *Learning Disabilities,* eds. N. N. Singh and I. L. Beale. New York: Springer-Verlag.

Strauss, A. A., and Lehtinen, L. E. 1947. *Psychopathology and Education of the Brain-injured Child.* New York: Grune & Stratton.

U. S. Department of Education, Office of Educational Research and Assessment. 1989. *Digest of Education Statistics.*

U. S. Office of Education. 1977, December 29. Assistance to the States for education of handicapped children. Procedures for evaluating specific learning disabilities. *Federal Register* 42(250):65082–85.

Walsh, E. A. 1914. Ungraded class work in New York City—methods and results. *Journal of Psycho-asthenics* 19:59–66.

Chapter • 2

Specific Reading Disability
Splitting and Lumping

Bruce K. Shapiro

Reading is essential for successful functioning within our society; it is the major means of information acquisition, and the foundation for employability. Level of literacy is correlated with economic status and is associated with income, ultimate vocation, and continued vocational flexibility. The importance of literacy to social function has increased over the past century. Failure to attain literacy is linked to adverse social outcomes, such as premature exit from school, teenaged pregnancy, juvenile delinquency, chronic welfare dependence, and drug abuse (Schonaut and Satz 1983). Remedial reading programs can be found in colleges, private industry, and the armed services. More recently, community-based programs designed to help adults attain the reading skills required for work and social function have received much support.

The past 30 years have seen explosive growth of specific reading disability in clinical and research areas. Despite an increasing number of children receiving special education for specific learning disorder, and intensive research into the etiology and treatment of this disorder, the number of children served with the diagnosis of specific reading disability continues to increase. Specific reading disorder is an example of a disability wherein the management preceded the research. It is only now that the precepts upon which the concept, specific reading disability, was established are being reexamined.

SPECIFIC READING DISABILITY: SYNDROME OR DISORDER?

The first level of splitting is the recognition that something is different from the population at large. This requires the observer to decide that the finding is meaningfully different and to develop criteria so that others may recognize it. In the case of specific reading disability, the salient features were outlined at the turn of the century (Hinshelwood 1917): (1) difficulty reading in (2) an individual who has sufficient intellect and (3) adequate instruction. These features still delineate the syndrome. The first characteristic was the hallmark of the syndrome— young adults who were not able to read. Sufficient intellect was a required characteristic that distinguished specific reading disability from mental retardation. Adequate instruction was relevant at the turn of the century when universal education was not the rule.

A syndrome's borders blur as they evolve. Cases that were not so clear as the initial descriptions are now included in the category. Criteria for definition may change and the methods used to define the syndrome may be modified. Specific reading disorder evolved from its earliest descriptions and encompassed larger populations as the construct developed. Hinshelwood felt that dyslexia was quite rare (Hinshelwood 1917). Orton suggested a number that was somewhat larger. Samuel Kirk was motivated by the need to serve a large number of children with substandard reading achievement and coined the term *specific learning disability*. He promulgated the discrepancy approach to diagnosis (Doris 1993). More recently, Shaywitz and co-workers (1990) postulated that specific reading disability was merely the end of the normal curve of reading disability.

SPECIFIC READING DISABILITY: IS THE CONSTRUCT STILL USEFUL?

As the number of children with specific reading disability has increased and as the number of different associations has been delineated, the concept of specific reading disability has come into question. One of the fundamental precepts of dyslexia is that affected children learn differently from children whose reading difficulty derives from low intellect. This latter group of children has been referred to as "garden variety" poor readers. Comparisons of the reading progress of "garden variety" poor readers and children with specific reading disability found that children with specific reading disability learned reading in a fashion not unlike that of slow readers (Stanovich 1994).

Another fundamental precept, that these children acquire reading skills at a rate that is disproportionate to their intellectual skills, has also been questioned in three different ways. Siegel and co-workers have challenged the use of IQ to develop discrepancy formulas that define specific reading disability (Siegel 1989). This argument is based on several factors. First, IQ and reading ability are dependent constructs; language abilities make substantial contributions to IQ and to reading. Second, IQ is not related to reading ability in a linear fashion. Third, reading difficulties may diminish the rate of intellectual growth and thereby obscure the discrepancy between reading ability and IQ.

The second question centers on whether reading acquisition is related to IQ in a continuous fashion, that is, that IQ should predict reading ability for the individual child. Taken to its extreme, the assumption of a continuous relationship allows bright children whose academic performance is above classroom expectations, but not above IQ expectations, to be classified as disabled. At the other end of the cognitive spectrum, dependence on a continuous relationship precludes the provision of special education to children who read poorly even though the long-term negative consequences are well known. An alternate position holds that a certain amount of intellect is required for reading, but that beyond the minimum, reading proceeds independent of a summary IQ. Those who advocate a threshold relationship strive to answer the question, "What is the minimum intellect required for the normal acquisition of reading skills?" Although there is a correlation between reading and IQ for populations, Share and co-workers (1989) have demonstrated in a population-based, epidemiological study that the relationship between intellect and reading ability is not linear for individual children. Some children whose IQs would predict "garden variety" poor readers, attain reading skills at significantly advanced rates.

Finally, several studies have challenged the ability of IQ-Achievement discrepancy formulas to appropriately identify children with specific reading disability. These studies have reported that children with specific reading disability are typically under identified by using discrepancy formulas (Forness 1983; Shapiro et al. 1990). Some of the reasons for this are: age of the child, severity of the reading dysfunction, test characteristics, and co-morbid developmental, behavioral, and emotional conditions (attention deficit hyperactivity disorder, developmental language disorder, affective disorders).

The initial reports of dyslexia focused on adults. It is not difficult to identify dyslexia in an adult. However, in young children, specific reading disability is not an easy diagnosis to make. Shaywitz and co-workers (Shaywitz et al.1990) followed a group of children, in a longitudinal fashion and found that children grew in and out of the diagnosis of specific reading disability. They suggested that specific reading disability is not a static diagnosis. Alternatively, the data may be interpreted to describe a heterogeneous population with similar early characteristics, but within that population are children who are temporarily delayed in the acquisition of reading skills: those whose reading skill acquisition is delayed because of a more generalized process; those who have lasting deficits; those whose deficits do not become apparent until the system is put to the test; and those who compensate for their deficits. Trying to distinguish which children are going to have *persisting* deficits among a general population of children is indeed difficult. It may not be possible to identify children with true disabilities apart from the larger group of children who are transiently poor readers. This is not to imply that factors associated with reading disability may be identified at an early age and remediated, but that it is likely that many children so treated will receive unnecessary remediation.

The early descriptions of dyslexia included failure to read despite adequate instruction because universal education was not assumed in the late nineteenth century. A small number of reports of large urban schools with generally low academic achievement have raised again the specter of instructional inadequacy instead of specific reading disability. Recent discussions of the relationship between instruction and academic success center on a variety of factors including teacher variables, time, curricular content, structural characteristics (class size, space configurations), readiness to learn, and family and social influences (Johnson 1994). Consequently, it is difficult to answer the question of whether instruction is adequate.

IS SPECIFIC READING DISABILITY A SINGLE ENTITY?

The rapid increase in the prevalence of specific reading disability may stem from several causes. An initial surge was expected in the early 1980s as school systems were charged to provide appropriate remediation for specific reading disability. The increase in specific reading disability has continued, however, and although the reasons for this are not clear, several hypotheses have been suggested. First, the prevalence is increasing; second, attempts to identify children at earlier ages result in over identification; and third, techniques used to classify specific reading disability may be faulty. Finally, the definition of specific reading disability may be expanding over time and may subsume related diagnoses such as mental retardation that seem to be decreasing over the same time span.

Reviewing the evolution of specific reading disability leads to the conclusion that specific reading disability is a syndrome and not a single disorder. (Children may meet diagnostic criteria as a result of differing etiologies.) Dyslexia, as defined by Hinshelwood, is but one of a group of specific reading *disabilities* that has been most closely associated with those children who evidence phonological disturbances (Catts 1996). Other specific reading disabilities may derive from low intellect that affects reading to a greater degree than other abilities, generalized language disorder (Bishop and Adams 1990), and children with a delayed maturation of phonetic awareness. Other reading disabilities have been noted in "overload" situations, as in attention deficit hyperactivity disorder, transitioning from page to chapter reading, and those whose slow reading rate adversely affects performance on timed tests. Whether a spatial form of specific reading disability exists is still debated (Bakker 1992).

STUDYING MECHANISMS OF READING DYSFUNCTION

Specific reading disability is a concept in a state of revision. Attempts to better understand children with reading dysfunctions lead to a reconceptualization of the disorders. Understanding the mechanism(s) of specific reading disability is desirable for several reasons. Perhaps the most important reason is that it will facilitate understanding. Current understanding is limited by our focus on reading dysfunction. Co-morbid conditions, such as other specific learning disabilities in mathematics and written expression; attention deficit hyperactivity disorder, particularly the inattentive form; depression; or motor coordination disorders may not represent the co-occurrence of separate disorders but manifestations of a single entity. Indeed, it may be that the definition of specific reading disability is too narrow!

The ability to define the mechanism of specific reading disability may provide a better view of compensatory and age dependent changes that alter the expression of this syndrome. Providing non-educational therapies could be possible, as could identification of children for whom there is no effective therapy at earlier ages. Knowledge of the mechanism of specific reading disability would likely enhance prognostication. If a mechanism of specific reading disability were known, precipitating causes could be identified and potentially prevented. On a broader level, the identification of the brain dysfunctions of specific reading disability may improve understanding of the more global dysfunctions associated with mental retardation and developmental language disorder.

69915

Ashland Community College

Many approaches have been used to define specific reading disability better. Until recently, the most common methods have focused upon the *clinical performances* of children and young adults with reading problems or dysfunction. Grouping by risk status, test performance, presumed mechanisms of dysfunction, and types of errors have been attempted. Test performance is a proxy for the clinical state. It is the main way that specific reading disability is defined at this time. The problem is that the tests are not "pure" and other functional difficulties (attention, language, motivation) influence test performance. Issues of test construction and measurement are significant. In addition, multiple samplings increase the chances that a child will demonstrate a deficit on a test, making it unlikely to find a child who is free of other factors. Using other criteria to define specific reading disability has similarly resulted in finding small numbers of "pure groups," the vast majority being "mixed." (See review of Hooper and Swartz 1994.)

Patterns of test performance are hypothesized to represent different neuropsychological processes. At the most unadorned level are those children who show lower verbal than performance IQ. Use of multivariate statistical techniques have defined multiple types of reading disability (Korhonen 1991; Shafrir and Siegel 1994). Deficient neuropsychological processes, while associated with poor reading, are not causal. Kinsbourne el al. (1991) noted persistence of neuropsychological dysfunctions in a group of adults who were diagnosed with specific reading disability, but who attained literacy. This finding raises the question as to whether the mechanism of specific reading disability is always associated with poor reading. If not, then the provocative factors remain to be discerned.

Some investigators have evaluated children with *known genetic syndromes* associated with specific reading disability, such as neurofibromatosis, and sought to find a "pure" form of specific reading disability (Udwin and Dennis 1995; Denckla 1996). The reading disability found in children with Neurofibromatosis Type 1 was broader than that seen in dyslexics and was more consistent with a more general language-based reading disorder. Inter-individual genetic differences, severity of reading dysfunction, cognitive variability, and degree of difference from control populations were among the factors posited to affect the ability to discern a mechanism.

Another means of selecting a population to study would be to evaluate children who exhibited *unresponsiveness to interventions* designed to treat/prevent specific reading disability. For example, Gillon and Dodd (1994) and Scanlon and Vellutino (1996) have both published studies optimistic about phonetic training. Despite their excellent results, there are still some children who have difficulties. This group would be worthy of further study.

Other authors have attempted to look at more "basic" processing functions. Some of these authors have dealt with more complex auditory (Tallal 1993; Merzenich et al. 1996) or visual abilities (Eden et al. 1995), while others have assessed more fundamental abilities and used psychophysical measures. These approaches are not so confounded as the more traditional clinical performance measures, but they are also more distant from the target behavior—reading. Consequently, it becomes more difficult to assign causality from any relationships that may be found.

More recently, physiologic approaches that quantify brain activation during the reading process have been applied to normal and dyslexic adults. Functional neuroimaging studies using a variety of techniques (PET, EEG, rCBF, fMRI) have shown differences between adults with reading disabilities and others (Rumsey et al. 1995; Kraus et al. 1996; Flowers et al. 1991; Eden et al. 1996). The studies have not yielded consistent findings, nor is it clear that the differences noted will be strong enough to be applied to individuals. If these studies are properly validated, they will represent a major advance over the anatomical reports that impute function based on structure.

Specific reading disability has long been thought to have a genetic substrate. Epidemiologic studies, twin studies, and linkage analyses have all pointed to heritable etiologies for some forms of specific reading disability (DeFries and Alarcon 1996). Some investigators have localized dyslexia to a small portion of chromosome 6 (Cardon et al. 1994,1995). Whether these cases are unique, or representative of the broader population of specific reading disability, awaits further study.

Current techniques to identify mechanisms proceed from a functional base and become increasingly unrelated to reading. While many associations have been delineated, causal relationships have not been established. The methods used are highly subject to artifact, and cross-subject comparisons are difficult. In the final analysis, group associations may be found, but they may not yield much useful information for individuals because their sensitivity and specificity may be too low for clinical use. A more frightening possibility is that knowing the mechanism may not achieve any of the objectives outlined above.

CLINICAL REALITY: ARE THERE PURE CASES?

Clinicians who treat children with specific reading disability are more often struck by the variety than the similarity. The diagnosis is simply the most obvious manifestation of the neurologic dysfunction. As is true of most children with developmental disorders, multiple diagnoses are the rule. Common co-morbid conditions include ADHD, psychiatric dysfunction (affective, anxiety, adjustment), language disorders, and fine motor dysfunction. The degree to which these disorders vary determines the clinical picture. The continuum of factors that must be considered when treating children with specific reading disorders is broad. In the final analysis, each child has his own individual disorder. "Pure" cases are the exception.

Successful treatment depends on understanding the patient within his or her context. Patient variables, diagnosis variables, family variables, school variables, and social variables all have an impact on the outcome of a proposed treatment program. The first thing to do is to establish all relevant diagnoses. Effective techniques for reading remediation may fail in the presence of insufficiently treated ADHD, language disorders, motor dysfunction, or psychiatric disorders (Kube and Shapiro (1996). In addition to the diagnoses, other important patient variables include: severity of dysfunction, temperament, self esteem, and motivation. School variables, including type of school, composition of student body, teachers' experience, and attitudes toward disabilities need to be considered. Indeed, for some children, these factors mandate a change in school. Family variables include number of parents, siblings, marital stability, parent rearing styles, parental education, and other family members with disabilities. Social variables include income, safety, housing, and access to resources. All must be considered when developing a treatment plan for an individual child.

Education is the keystone of therapy for the child with specific reading disability and there are many approaches—top down, bottom up, information processing theory, and interactive theories. Most teachers prefer an eclectic multisensory approach to remediation. While some choose to bypass weaknesses and circumvent the reading disorder by non-print means, others use some circumvention techniques (readers, tapes, videos, group activities) to insure that impaired reading ability does not become a generalized disability. Similar options exist in the management of other aspects of specific reading disability.

CLINICAL SPLITTING AND RESEARCH LUMPING OR VICE VERSA

The goals of the research and clinical approaches to specific reading disability are the same: improved outcomes. Research and clinical management are inextricably linked, complementary functions that result in improved care of children with specific reading disability. Neither can exist in the absence of the other. Ideally, clinical questions motivate research, and the principles derived from research lead to improved outcomes. In the best situation, research leads to prevention or cure; failing that, to improved management. Despite identical goals, the approaches used in research and clinical care are markedly different.

These differences may lead to misunderstanding and the devaluation of one approach or the other. Inexperienced researchers stereotype clinicians as sloppy, clumpers, or ancecdotal, and view themselves as scientific, rigorous, and precise. Nihilistic clinicians dismiss research as irrelevant. There is a need to bridge the gap between clinical and research approaches. Understanding the limits of each approach will improve the care of children with specific reading disability. Perhaps the differences are illustrated by the following two examples.

The first example comes from a study published in the *Journal of Learning Disabilities* (Eden et al. 1995).

> Reading Disability (RD). Selected from the poor reading sample, this group's reading score at fifth grade on the WJRSS was below 85. Like the normally achieving group's their IQs on the WISC-R were between 85 and 115. (p. 274)

The second is abstracted from a clinical case report.

> Richard is a 7.5 year old who has been referred for academic and behavior problems in school. He is having difficulty paying attention in his 2nd grade class. His reading abilities are poor and he is beginning to withdraw socially. Richard's problems are not new. He has had reports of poor attention since beginning school. Richard is not learning to read. His teacher says Richard does not know the names of all the lower-case letters and he doesn't know the sounds of most letters. He "reads" by guessing based on the configurations of the words. Richard spends two hours a night trying to do his homework. His mother reports that he is unable to do his homework independently. Richard was evaluated by the school team at the end of first grade and found eligible to receive special education services. Richard's mother did not want him "labeled," nor did she want him coming into contact with the "wrong sort." His current class consists of a teacher and 35 children with a wide range of abilities. There are four other children in Richard's class who are receiving special education services using a "pull out" model.

The goals are the same but research and clinical care have different foci, objectives, and benefits. Research focuses on the disorder in isolation of other factors. The clinical approach focuses on the individual. Research attempts to define "pure" groups in order to identify general principles and determine the mechanism of dysfunction. Clinical approaches apply general principles to specific cases. Research tries to minimize the number of operational variables to discern effects.

Table I.   Comparison of Clinical and Research Approaches

	Clinical Approach	Research Approach
Goal	Improved outcomes	Improved outcomes
Focus	Individual	Disorder
Objectives	Apply general principles to specific cases	Determine mechanism of dysfunction
	Current, intermediate, long-term approaches	Identify general principles
Outcomes	Academic	Diagnosis
	Vocational	Prognosis
	Social	Treatment
	Emotional	Prevention

In specific reading disability, this is extremely difficult. Some cases may be "pure" but they are in the minority. Furthermore, external factors may significantly influence the treatment of an individual.

The clinical questions to be addressed by research are well established. Is there a way of preventing specific reading disability? Who is going to develop specific reading disability? What is the best way of treating it? Can we forecast what this child's reading ability will be when he is an adult? Much of the current research focuses on a means of delineating the syndrome that will allow it to be defined independently of the defining characteristic—poor reading. Other efforts are directed at finding effective treatment and management strategies.

Proper clinical approaches take a longitudinal view. Understanding current, immediate, and long-term aspects of the disorders are required to develop a comprehensive clinical management plan. Failure to consider long-term goals and objectives frequently results in unsuccessful outcomes. Research may be cross-sectional, limited to a single point in time, or longitudinal.

Both clinical and research approaches lump and split. Research tries to split the population into meaningful groups and discern principles that will apply to a group (lump). Clinical approaches use general principles to develop individualized management plans for heterogeneous populations (split). There will be no progress in specific reading disability unless both approaches are used.

REFERENCES

Bakker, D. J. 1992. Neuropsychological classification and treatment of dyslexia. *Journal of Learning Disabilities* 25:102–9.

Bishop, D. V. J. and Adams, C. 1990. A prospective study of the relationship between specific language impairment, phonological disorders, and reading retardation. *Journal of Child Psychology and Psychiatry* 31:1027–50.

Cardon, L. R., Smith, S. D., Fulker, D. W., Kimberling, W. J., Pennington, B. F., and DeFries, J. C. 1995. Quantitative trait locus for reading disability on chromosome 6. *Science* 266:276–79.

Cardon, L. R., Smith, S. D., Fulker, D. W., Kimberling, W. J., Pennington, B. F., and DeFries, J. C. 1995. Quantitative trait locus for reading disability: Correction (letter). *Science* 268:1553.

Catts, H. W. 1996. Defining dyslexia as a developmental language disorder: An expanded view. *Topics in Language Disorders* 16:14–29.

DeFries, J. C. and Alarcon, M. 1996. Genetics of specific reading disability. *Mental Retardation and Developmental Disabilities Research Reviews* 2:39–47.

Denckla, M. B. 1996. Neurofibromatosis Type 1: A model for the pathogenesis of reading disability. *Mental Retardation and Developmental Disabilities Research Reviews* 2:48–53.

Doris, J. L. 1993. Defining learning disabilities. A history of the search for consensus. In *Better Understanding of Learning Disabilities*, eds. G. R. Lyon, D. B. Gray, J. F. Kavanagh, and N. A. Krasnegor. Baltimore: Brookes.

Eden, G. F., Stein, J. F.,Wood, M. H., and Wood, F. B. 1995. Verbal and visual problems in reading disability. *Journal of Learning Disabilities* 28:272–90.

Eden, G. F., VanMeter, J. W., Rumsey, J. M., Maisog, J. M., Woods, R. P., and Zeffiro, T. A. 1996. Abnormal processing of visual motion in dyslexia revealed by functional brain imaging. *Nature* 382:66–69.

Flowers, D. L., Wood, F. B., and Naylor, C. E. 1991. Regional cerebral blood flow correlates of language processes in reading disability. *Archives of Neurology* 48:637–43.

Forness, S. R., Sinclair, E., and Guthrie, D. 1983. Learning disability discrepancy formulas: Their uses in actual practice. *Learning Disability Quarterly* 6:107–14.

Gillon, G., and Dodd, B. 1994. The effects of training phonological, semantic, and syntactic processing skills in spoken language on reading ability. *Reading and Writing* 6:321–45.

Hinshelwood, J. 1917. *Congenital Word Blindness*. Chicago: Medical Book Co.

Hooper, S. R., and Swartz, C. 1994. Learning Disability Subtypes. Splitting versus lumping revisited. In *Learning Disability Spectrum: ADD, ADHD, and LD*, eds. A. J. Capute, P. J. Accardo, and B. K. Shapiro. Baltimore: York Press.

Johnson, D. J. 1994. Educational interventions in learning disabilities. Follow-up studies and future research needs. In *Learning Disability Spectrum: ADD, ADHD, and LD*, eds. A. J. Capute, P. J. Accardo, and B. K. Shapiro. Baltimore: York Press.

Kinsbourne, M., Rufo, D. T., Gamzu, E., Palmer, R. L., and Berliner, A. K. 1991. Neuropsychological deficits in adults with dyslexia. *Developmental Medicine and Child Neurology* 33:763–75.

Korhonen, T. T. 1991. An empirical subgrouping of Finnish learning-disabled children. *Journal of Clinical and Experimental Neuropsychology* 13:259–77.

Kraus, N., McGee, T. J., Carrell, T. D., Zecker, S. G., Nicol, T. G., and Koch, D. B. 1996. Auditory neurophysiologic responses and discrimination deficits in children with learning problems. *Science* 273:971–73.

Kube, D. A., and Shapiro, B. K. 1996. Persistent school dysfunction: Unrecognized comorbidity and suboptimal therapy. *Clinical Pediatrics* 35:571–76.

Merzenich, M. M., Jenkins, W. M., Johnston, P., Schreiner, C., Miller, S. L., and Tallal, P. 1996. Temporal processing deficits of language-learning impaired children ameliorated by training. *Science* 271:77–80.

Rumsey, J. M., Nace, K., and Andreason, P. 1995. Phonologic and ortho-graphic components of reading imaged with PET. *Journal of the International Neuropsychological Society* 1:180.

Scanlon, D. M., and Vellutino, F. R. 1996. Prerequisite skills, early instruction, and success in first- grade reading: Selected results from a longitudinal study. *Mental Retardation and Developmental Disabilities Research Reviews* 2:54–63.

Schonaut, S., and Satz, P. 1983. Prognosis for children with learning disabilities: A review of follow-up studies. In *Developmental Neuropsychiatry*, ed. M. Rutter. New York: The Guilford Press.

Shafrir, U., and Siegel, L. S. 1994. Subtypes of learning disabilities in adoles-cents and adults. *Journal of Learning Disabilities* 27:123–34.

Shapiro, B. K., Palmer, F. B., Antell, S. E., Bilker, S., Ross, A., and Capute, A. J. 1990. Detection of young children in need of reading help. Evaluation of specific reading disability formulas. *Clinical Pediatrics* 29:206–13.

Share, D. L., McGee, R., and Silva, P. A. 1989. IQ and reading progress: A test of the capacity notion of IQ. *Journal of the American Academy of Child and Adolescent Psychiatry* 28:97–100.

Shaywitz, S. E., Escobar, M. D., Shaywitz, B. A., Fletcher, J. M., and Makuch, R. R. 1990. Evidence that dyslexia may represent the lower tail of a normal distribution of reading ability. *New England Journal of Medicine* 326:145–50.

Siegel, L. S. 1989. IQ is irrelevant to the definition of Learning Disabilities. *Journal of Learning Disabilities* 22:469–78.

Stanovich, K. E. 1994. Annotation: Does Dyslexia Exist? *Journal of Child Psychology and Psychiatry* 35:579–95.

Tallal, P., Miller, S., and Fitch, R. H. 1993. Neurobiological basis of the case for the preeminence of temporal processing. In *Temporal Information Processing in the Nervous System: Special Reference to Dyslexia and Dysphasia*, eds. P. Tallal, A. M. Galaburda, R. R. Llinás, and C. von Euler. New York: The New York Academy of Sciences.

Udwin, O., and Dennis, J. 1995. Psychological and behavioural phenotypes in genetically determined syndromes: A review of research findings. In *Behavioural Phenotypes*, eds. G. O'Brien, and W. Yule. London: MacKeith Press.

Section • II

Mechanisms of Specific Reading Disability

Chapter • 3

Functional Neuroimaging of Developmental Dyslexia
Regional Cerebral Blood Flow in Dyslexic Men

Judith M. Rumsey and
Guinevere Eden

Functional neuroimaging provides a window through which to capture a glimpse of brain activity. The development of techniques for imaging physiological processes, such as the changes in cerebral blood flow that accompany neuronal activity, has made it possible to view the brain at work. Both positron emission tomography (PET) and, more recently, functional magnetic resonance imaging (fMRI), have begun to provide noninvasive techniques for determining task-related changes in regional cerebral blood flow both in healthy individuals and in patients. These techniques can be used to map the brain regions and pathways involved in normal cognitive activity and to probe the integrity of these regions and pathways in developmental disorders.

Functional neuroimaging holds particular promise for the study of developmental disorders. Until recently, inferences about brain function in developmental disorders were generally based on neuropsychological tests validated in patients (usually adults) with acquired (as opposed to congenital) brain lesions. Tests designed to capture deficits seen in such patients may be limited in their sensitivity to the more subtle deficits that characterize developmental disorders. Furthermore, given their early (prenatal) onset, the neuropathology associated with developmental disorders impacts brain structure and functions in ways that are poorly understood, but which is likely to differ in its impact from that associated with acquired pathology. Neuroimaging now provides an unprecedented opportunity to more directly examine brain function in dyslexia and other developmental disorders.

This chapter describes the first studies of regional cerebral blood flow in developmental dyslexia that have used state-of-the-art neuroimaging techniques—namely, positron emission tomography (PET) and functional magnetic resonance imaging (fMRI). These studies have examined task-related alterations in blood flow, or blood oxygenation, which themselves are indirect reflections of neuronal activity, in a carefully selected sample of men with persisting reading deficits due to developmental dyslexia. The neural correlates of both language-related and visual processing abnormalities were assessed in these studies.

DIAGNOSTIC ISSUES AND SAMPLE SELECTION

Definitions of developmental dyslexia vary in their inclusiveness and are still evolving. While some definitions (American Psychiatric Association 1994) include deficits in reading comprehension, most focus on deficits in word recognition or reading decoding—the ability to read words accurately and fluently—as the core defining feature. Indeed, reading comprehension, while constrained by deficits in decoding (Conners and Olson 1990), is generally better than that expected on the basis of decoding skills, consistent with intact spoken language comprehension in many or most dyslexic individuals (Bishop and Adams, 1990). Indeed, some researchers have argued for definitions that incorporate discrepancies between relatively intact language comprehension (i.e., listening comprehension) and reading decoding. Such definitions would exclude children with developmental language disorders, whose poor reading reflects deficits in the comprehension of spoken language (Bishop and Adams 1990).

Deficits in reading rate and fluency have been afforded less attention than have those in reading accuracy. Indeed, few standardized psychometric tests of reading skill include timed measures of the ability to read connected text aloud. When clinically evaluating adolescents and adults with histories of dyslexia, it is not uncommon to see individuals who score well on untimed tests of single word recognition, such as the Woodcock-Johnson tests, but who read so slowly that they remain significantly impaired. This slowness is not captured or reflected in the scores generated with most reading tests, thus complicating the diagnosis of dyslexia in adolescents and adults. A rare exception is the Gray Oral Reading Test-3rd edition (GORT-3), a timed test of oral paragraph reading (Wiederholt and Bryant 1992).

Finally, until recently, dyslexia was diagnosed only in the presence of a significant discrepancy between general intelligence, as measured by IQ, and reading skill (American Psychiatric Association 1994). However, because recent studies have shown that the phonological deficits associated with poor reading skill are similar in individuals with high and with low IQ scores (Siegel 1992; Stanovich and Siegel 1994), some researchers now advocate a definition based on poor reading regardless of level of general intelligence. Such a definition would include individuals with low IQ scores. While strong associations between phonological deficits and poor reading may reflect a causative relationship with implications for intervention, relationships between IQ and brain size (Andreasen et al. 1993) are consistent with the hypothesis that brain structure and possibly function differ in individuals with high versus low general intelligence. Thus, for purposes of brain imaging research, it is probably best to study dyslexic subjects with average versus low IQ scores as separate groups.

The functional imaging studies described in this chapter employed a conservative definition of dyslexia; that is, the individuals studied, all of whom were men, were selected so that most, if not all, researchers would agree with their diagnosis as dyslexic. All had childhood histories of developmental reading disorder, continued to show at least mild deficits in decoding (when using measures of timed oral paragraph reading), and had at least average intelligence (Eden et al. 1996; Rumsey et al. 1997). Their reading comprehension and verbal comprehension skills were good. In addition, they performed poorly on measures of phonological processing, including tests of phonological awareness and pseudoword reading (see Eden et al. 1996 and Rumsey et al. 1997). The reason for limiting these studies to men was the fact that more males have historically been identified as reading disabled, although recent epidemiological research (Shaywitz et al. 1990) suggests that nearly as many females are affected. Nonetheless, to recruit an adequate number of subjects with clear childhood diagnoses, it was practically necessary to selectively focus on males because of this historical trend.

NEUROBEHAVIORAL DEFICITS IN DYSLEXIA

Children learn to read via several interrelated mechanisms. They learn to recognize visual patterns—letter sequences and whole words—through experience (Ehri and Wilce 1985). The term "orthographic" has been applied to this process, which involves both visual analysis and the recognition of spelling patterns (Vellutino et al. 1995). They also learn to "sound out" words by applying phonological rules for relating letters and letter combination (graphemes) to speech sounds (phonemes) (Wagner and Torgesen 1987). This phonological component involves the use of the speech code to store and retrieve information (Vellutino et al. 1995). Words are segmented into sublexical units (syllables; "onsets" or beginning consonants; and "rimes" or vowel-consonant combinations; individual phonemes), and their speech sound representations are accessed and combined, or blended. Finally, children also learn new words by applying what they know about words in their reading vocabulary to new, unfamiliar words; that is, they "read by analogy" to known words (Goswami 1986).

In dyslexia, some of these mechanisms fail. While the neuropsychological deficits associated with dyslexia vary from individual to individual, behavioral research has made a solid case for phonological deficits causing the word recognition deficits that characterize dyslexia. Phonological awareness in young preschool-age children is predictive of success in learning to read (Liberman and Shankweiler, 1985; Wagner and Torgesen, 1987). Furthermore, training to improve phonological awareness results in improved word recognition (Blachman 1991; Bradley and Bryant 1983; Brady and Shankweiler 1991). While young dyslexic children show deficits in both phonological and orthographic components of reading skill, as they mature, those who improve their reading do so primarily by improving their orthographic skills (Olson et al. 1989). Phonological deficits persist even into adulthood (Olson et al. 1989; Pennington et al. 1987), making it possible to study these deficits in dyslexic adults.

Other neuropsychological deficits are seen in dyslexia, but their role and relationship to word recognition deficits may differ from those associated with core phonological deficits. Deficits in rapid naming may contribute independently to slow, inefficient reading of connected text (Bowers and Wolf 1993). Associated language deficits, such as those in syntax, semantics and verbal memory may accompany the phonological deficits (Brady 1986; Mann and Brady 1988; Satz and Morris 1981), but their contributions to reading success or failure are less clear. Deficits in rapid temporal processing within the auditory system have also been hypothesized (Tallal et al. 1993). The nature of such deficits and their role in reading require further study, however (Studdert-Kennedy and Mody 1995). Finally, deficits in visuospatial memory and learning are seen less frequently, and the view that they contribute to dyslexia has been largely refuted. (See Willows 1991.)

With the use of psychophysical methods, other specific visual processing abnormalities involving the early processing of temporal sequences of stimuli in dyslexia have been identified. The ability to discriminate stimuli presented in rapid temporal succession has been shown to be deficient. Visual persistence (the duration during which an image is perceived even after the removal of a stimulus) has been found to be prolonged in reading disabled children (Stanley et al. 1983). Visual persistence can be assessed by presenting two separate stimuli in close succession and determining the point at which the two stimuli are perceived as one. Using such methods, reading disabled children have been found to have significantly longer separation thresholds (Stanley et al. 1983).

Using a technique in which subjects judged a grating stimulus, consisting of black and white bars, Lovegrove and Brown (1978) varied the spatial frequency of the stimulus (the number of lines within a space, with many lines resulting in a high spatial frequency) and measured the effect on the subject's perception. In adults, the duration of visual persistence increases as spatial frequency increases (as the gratings become less coarse). Lovegrove and colleagues found this increase or function to be reduced in reading disabled children compared to normal control children (Lovegrove et al. 1980). Therefore, at low spatial frequencies (coarse gratings), reading disabled children exhibited longer visual persistence. In addition, when contrast (the luminance difference between light and dark bars) was reduced, reading disabled children were less able than controls to perceive the gratings (Martin and Lovegrove 1984).

Because information about contrast, spatial frequency and temporal properties are differentially processed within the visual system, these findings suggested dysfunction limited to a specific subsystem. Lovegrove et al. (1980) explained these findings within the framework of the sustained and transient channels of the visual pathway (Lovegrove 1993), sometimes referred to as the parvocellular and magnocellular systems, respectively. These channels are distinguished by their spatial frequency preference (for thick versus thin alternating black and white bars), their temporal properties and their contrast sensitivity. As summarized in figure 1, the neurons in the magnocellular layers of the lateral geniculate nucleus of the thalamus respond to stimuli with lower contrast, or smaller differences between the grayness of a dark and a light bar, compared to those neurons in the parvocellular layers. Because sensitivity to contrast, spatial frequency, and visual persistence were abnormal in reading disabled children, Lovegrove hypothesized a dysfunctional transient system, which mediates global form, movement, and temporal resolution. Consistent with this hypothesis, experiments in which flicker thresholds were used to measure the efficiency of the transient system successfully differentiated normal and reading disabled children (Martin and Lovegrove 1988). Flicker thresholds are determined by having individuals adjust the contrast level of a grating stimulus at different rates of flicker until they perceive a striped pattern. While such deficits in transient visual processing have not been causally linked to poor reading, it has been proposed that such an abnormality might prevent the uptake of crucial information required for the formation of spelling to sound correspondences (Breitmeyer 1980). However, there is no direct evidence to support this.

Unlike studies of language, studies of human visual processing have benefitted from a detailed understanding of underlying anatomy and physiology gained from experiments with non-human primates, which have yielded schemes for the functional specialization of the visual cortical pathways (Ungerleider and Mishkin 1982; Van Essen and Maunsell 1983). More recently, functional neuroimaging in humans utilizing PET and fMRI have identified a specific motion sensitive area, V5 or MT, in extrastriate cortex (Corbetta et al. 1990; Tootell et al. 1995; Watson et al. 1993), thought to be dominated by input from the magnocellular stream. (See figure 1.) The behavioral abnormalities identified in dyslexia associated with transient/magnocellular processing led Eden et al. (1996) to study this region of extrastriate cortex with fMRI in dyslexic men.

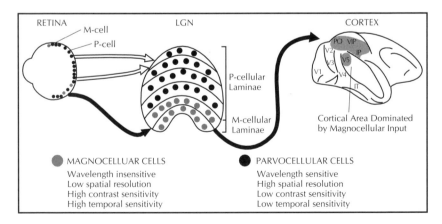

Figure 1. Functional specialization of the nonhuman primate visual system (adapted from Walsh 1995).

UNDERLYING NEUROPATHOLOGY

Given the limited availability of postmortem tissue in non-life-threatening disorders, few dyslexic brains have been autopsied. The studies of Galaburda and his colleagues represent the major work in this area. Because the functional imaging studies described in this chapter were limited to males, pathological findings in the male brains studied to date are most relevant here. Four consecutive male brains studied by Galaburda et al. (1985) showed developmental anomalies of the cerebral cortex, consisting of neuronal ectopias (displaced neurons) and architectonic dysplasias (distortions of the normal organized layering of the cortex). These anomalies, which appeared to be of prenatal origin, were seen on both sides of the brain, but showed a predilection for left perisylvian language cortex. Given that early lesions are capable of affecting developing connections between different cortical regions, Galaburda et al. (1985) hypothesized that they might impair brain function either directly and/or by forming improper connections. Thus, these congenital lesions might impair reading by rendering dysfunctional those brain regions which are critical to reading and/or by disconnecting them from other brain regions involved in language and visual processing. The variability in lesion distribution noted among the individual brains might also provide a basis for the variability in associated neuropsychological deficits seen in dyslexia.

Also reported in these brains were developmental anomalies within the lateral geniculate nucleus, a thalamic nucleus through which visual information is transmitted to the cortex (Livingstone et al. 1991). This structure consists of two ventral magnocellular (large-celled) layers and four dorsal parvocellular (small-celled) layers. (See figure 1.) Consistent with this anatomic segregation, single cell recordings in animals (Kaplan and Shapley 1982; Schiller and Colby 1983) have indicated that the magnocellular neurons respond only briefly, or "transiently," and with greater sensitivity to low contrast stimuli, while those neurons in the parvocellular layers, which preferentially subserve visual processing of structural detail and color, respond more to high contrast stimuli and exhibit a physiologically prolonged or "sustained" response. The outputs of these layers are thought to remain partially segregated as they project to higher-level extrastriate cortical areas involved in processing color and form versus motion (Ungerleider and Mishkin 1982). While the parvocellular layers of the lateral geniculate nucleus appeared normal in the dyslexic brains, the magnocellular layers were disorganized and the cell bodies within these layers appeared smaller in dyslexic than in the control brains (Livingstone et al. 1991). These findings were consistent with the hypothesis that deficits in rapid temporal visual processing in dyslexia result from a dysfunctional magnocellular visual system.

THE FUNCTIONAL NEUROANATOMY OF READING

Traditional models of the functional neuroanatomy of reading based on lesion studies (Henderson 1986) postulate that visual processing for reading occurs in striate (primary visual) and extrastriate (visual association) cortex in the occipital lobe. (See figure 2.) Information from both left and right visual cortex is transmitted to the left angular gyrus, which caps the posterior extent of the superior temporal sulcus. Information from the right occipital lobe is transmitted to the left side of the brain via commissural fibers that pass through the splenium (the bulbous, most posterior portion) of the corpus callosum. The left angular gyrus in the inferior parietal lobe appears to be crucial to reading and may be involved in translating written language into speech sound representations. Damage limited to the left angular gyrus or lesions that undercut its underlying white matter, thereby disconnecting it from other visual and language regions, disrupt reading without impairing spoken language. Further processing for meaning is thought to involve Wernicke's area in the left posterior superior temporal gyrus. In addition to this superior pathway through the left angular gyrus, inferior portions of the left temporal lobe may also play a significant role in reading. Wernicke's area projects to Broca's area in the left inferior frontal lobe. Broca's area is involved in articulatory and syntactic coding (Mesulam 1990). Connections among these cortical regions are generally bi–directional (Mesulam 1990). Thus, not only does Wernicke's area send connections forward to Broca's area, but Broca's area also sends projections back into Wernicke's area. These bi–directional connections provide for the simultaneous activity of these regions during reading and language processing.

Acquired brain lesions may differentially disrupt phonological and orthographic components of word recognition. Surface, or orthographic, alexics are impaired in their ability to read words with irregular spellings, but show a preserved ability to read regular words and pseudowords, demonstrating relatively intact phonological skills. Conversely, phonological alexics are unable to read pseudowords, but are relatively able to read real words; their orthographic skills are intact. Such dissociations have stimulated "dual-route" models of reading (Coltheart et al. 1993), which hypothesize the existence of independent neural pathways and distinctly different mechanisms subserving orthographic and phonological components of word

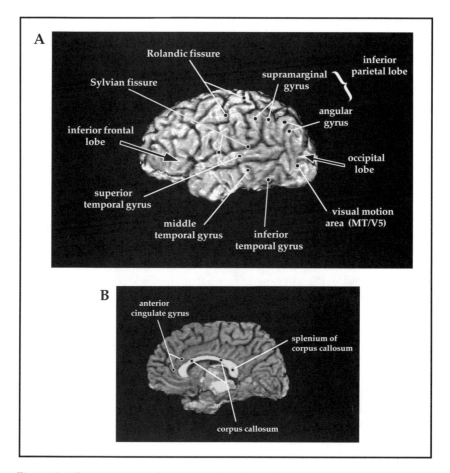

Figure 2.   Brain regions of interest in functional imaging studies of dyslexia.

recognition. Some researchers (McCarthy and Warrington 1990) have hypothesized that the critical lesion in phonological alexia resides in the left temporoparietal regions, while that in surface alexia lies in the left posterior temporal lobe. Attempts to establish distinctive neuroanatomical correlates of these syndromes, however, have been unsuccessful (Friedman et al. 1993). As an alternative to dual route models, single-route connectionist models of reading have proposed that both types of processing occur simultaneously in distributed neural networks (Plaut et al. 1996; Seidenberg and McClelland 1989). Within these models, both words and pseudowords are processed via a single interactive process and are represented as patterns of activations within local neural networks.

FUNCTIONAL NEUROIMAGING METHODS: PET AND fMRI

Positron emission tomography (PET), which became available in the 1980s, is a research technique that is useful for providing images of brain function. PET involves the injection of a radioactive tracer into an arm vein. The tracer is taken up by the brain in proportion to the degree of activity in specific brain regions. A ring of detectors around the subject's head measures the radioactivity and localizes its source within the brain, and the PET scanner constructs an image reflecting this information. A variety of physiological processes can be measured using PET. Most useful for measuring task-related cognitive activity are studies using oxygen-15-labelled water as a tracer to measure changes in regional cerebral blood flow. Current PET scanners, such as that used in the studies described below, have a spatial resolution on the order of 5mm and a temporal resolution on the order of 15 to 60 seconds. Spatial resolution refers to the distance at which two sources of radioactivity can be discerned as separate. Temporal resolution refers to the amount of time reflected in the images obtained from a single scan.

Functional magnetic resonance imaging (fMRI) became available in the 1990s. fMRI uses conventional MRI scanners together with fast imaging techniques to detect task-related signal changes related to blood flow and blood volume. Because it involves no ionizing radiation, it is safe for use with children. Furthermore, the data obtained generally are more easily interpretable for individual subjects than is data obtained with PET. Spatial resolution is on the order of 3mm; and temporal resolution, potentially superior to that of PET. Temporal resolution is, however, limited by the physiological response of the blood flow change, which occurs with an approximate six–second–delay following a stimulus. Anatomic scans obtained in the same scanning session can readily be coregistered with the functional scans, thus enhancing the match between brain structure and function for individual subjects. Additional descriptions of these techniques are found in Krasuski et al. (1996) and in Eden and Zeffiro (1996).

To identify regions involved in the performance of a task in imaging studies, two scans are compared. Fairly neutral control scans may provide a baseline against which to demonstrate the multiple regions activated by a task and to contrast the activations seen across tasks. To isolate the specific brain regions involved in a cognitive operation or mental function, scans acquired during the performance of tasks, which are identical save for one element or operation, are needed.

Auditory studies

The first PET studies of regional cerebral blood flow in dyslexia were published in the early 1990s (Rumsey et al. 1992; 1994a, b). These studies examined a group of 15 men with persistent developmental dyslexia (as described above). Controls were 20 healthy men with no history of developmental disorder who scored within a normal range on tests of reading, spelling and math achievement, as well as on tests of general intelligence. Auditory tasks which required no reading were used to minimize the contributions of reading deficits to any physiological abnormalities that might be seen in dyslexic men.

A variety of tasks were designed to probe left-sided language regions and homologous right-sided brain regions. The tasks were selected based on their neuropsychological relevance to dyslexia and prior neuroimaging findings indicating that the tasks would engage localized brain regions of interest in dyslexia. All the tasks used involved examiner-paced auditory presentations of paired items, decisions about whether or not the items within a pair matched each other in some way, and button press responses. For these early studies, each task was compared to a common resting baseline, during which subjects performed no task. The focus was on group comparisons. The major question was whether dyslexic men would normally activate left-sided language regions and their right-sided homologues during the performance of language and nonlanguage tasks expected to activate these regions in control men.

Because lack of phonological awareness, sometimes operationalized with rhyme detection tasks, is thought to cause reading deficits, a rhyme detection task was adapted for use with PET. The subjects listened to pairs of words and indicated with a button press those pairs that rhymed. As expected on the basis of other imaging work (Knopman et al. 1982; Petersen et al. 1989), this task activated in controls left temporoparietal cortex, as well as left posterior superior cortex (Rumsey et al. 1992). A syntax task required subjects to listen to paired sentences differing in grammatical structures and to press a button to indicate which pairs consisted of sentences with the same meaning. For example, the subject heard, "I'll go if you need me" and "Should you need me, I'll go." This task activated more anterior language regions in control men, including the left anterior temporal lobe and left inferior frontal lobe (Rumsey et al. 1994a, b), consistent with the involvement of Broca's area (in the left inferior frontal region) in syntactic coding (Mesulam 1990).

Because homologous right-sided regions were also of interest, a tonal memory task, shown previously to engage these regions (Mazziotta et al. 1982), was also adapted for use with PET (Rumsey et al. 1994a). In this task, subjects listened to paired sequences of three to four tones and indicated those pairs containing identical tone sequences. This task activated right frontotemporal regions in controls and thus provided a probe for the functional integrity of these regions in dyslexia.

Comparisons of the dyslexic men to their controls yielded several interesting findings: (1) At rest, the dyslexic men showed reduced blood flow only in the left inferior parietal lobe, near the angular and supramarginal gyri (Rumsey et al. 1994b). This focal reduction in blood flow was equal in magnitude to the task-related activations seen in controls and thus might reflect differences in functional activity associated with the resting state and/or disordered cytoarchitecture or other microscopic structural abnormalities reported in autopsy studies. (2) During the phonological, rhyme detection task, the dyslexic group failed to activate left temporoparietal cortex and left posterior superior temporal regions, regions activated by the control group during the performance of this task (Rumsey et al. 1992). (3) In contrast, dyslexic men showed robust and normal activation of the left inferior frontal regions during their performance of the syntax (sentence comprehension) task (Rumsey et al. 1994b). (4) During the tonal memory task, the dyslexic group showed reduced activation of right frontotemporal regions, showing significant activation of fewer regions than did their control singular group (Rumsey et al. 1994a). Performance by the dyslexic group on this latter nonlinguistic task, which was fast paced and difficult for both groups, was surprisingly impaired relative to their controls, indicating that the neuropsychological deficits of the dyslexic group extended beyond the processing of speech sounds.

While relationships between poor performance on a tonal memory task and reading deficits may be indirect, this task revealed additional significant differences in the dyslexics' activation of right-sided brain regions. Thus, task-related activation of both left and right temporal lobe regions, as well as left temporoparietal regions was reduced in dyslexia. In contrast, left inferior frontal language regions were activated normally by the dyslexic men. In summary, men with persisting reading deficits showed bilateral posterior abnormalities, but normal activation of anterior language regions in the left hemisphere. Their performance of a phonological awareness task was associated with a failure to activate normally the left temporoparietal cortex.

Mapping visual word recognition

To extend these findings and determine whether their localization was convergent with abnormalities seen during word recognition, a new study (reported in Rumsey et al. 1997a, b) was designed. Because phonological components of word recognition are thought to be disproportionately impaired in older individuals with dyslexia, this study sought to compare phonological and orthographic components of word recognition (1) to determine whether these components involved different neural pathways and (2) to localize the neural correlates of impaired word recognition and phonological deficits in dyslexia.

This study again examined a sample of men with clear childhood histories of dyslexia, at least average intelligence, and persistent reading deficits. Because the tasks designed for this study involved word recognition, the criterion of "persistent reading deficit" was operationalized using a measure of timed oral paragraph reading (the GORT-3)—a more sensitive measure of reading deficit than provided by tests of single word recognition. Indeed, approximately half of the dyslexic men selected for this study had single word recognition scores, as measured with the Wide Range Achievement Test-3rd edition (WRAT-3), within an average range.

PET was used to measure regional cerebral blood flow during the performance of several tasks. Two different types of word recognition tasks were employed to contrast phonological and orthographic coding. *Pronunciation* was used to contrast the reading aloud of irregular/inconsistent words (cocoa, bury) with the reading of pseudowords (cazot, bivy). The reading aloud of words with irregular spellings and/or inconsistent pronunciations engages *orthographic* processing because such words violate phonological rules and are recognized based on experience. The reading aloud of pseudowords engages phonological coding mechanisms and pathways since these items are novel and must be decoded or "sounded out" by applying phonological rules.

Other imaging studies which have compared real word and pseudoword reading (e.g., Nobre et al. 1994; Petersen et al. 1990) have failed to find differences between the two in activation. These studies have either created their pseudowords by changing a single letter of a real word, thus increasing the probability of the pseudowords being read by analogy to real words, or failed to describe the pseudowords used. Furthermore, such studies have not attended to the effects of word frequency, and effects of spelling regularity are seen only at low frequencies. Thus, to maximize the differences in the types of processing required for the two pronunciation tasks, only low frequency (uncommon) items were used. To decrease the probability of subjects' reading by analogy, pseudowords were created from low frequency rime units, i.e., unusual, infrequent vowel-consonant combinations, rather than from real words.

In addition, to differentially engage these types of processing, two *lexical decision making* tasks, designed by Olson et al. (1994) to segregate these components of word recognition in studies of dyslexia, were adapted to the imaging situation. The *phonological decision* task required the subject to indicate with a button press which of two pseudowords, closely matched for initial consonant and length (bape - baik, criel - cride), sounded like a real word. This task required the sounding out of unfamiliar pseudowords and decision making based on sound. The *orthographic decision* task required the subject to indicate which of two items, a word and its pseudohomophone (hoal - hole, coyn - coin), was a real word. Subjects were encouraged to respond as rapidly as possible, a strategy which encourages decision making based on the visual recognition of spelling patterns. Furthermore, because the two items within each pair shared the same pronunciation, these orthographic decisions had to reflect recognition of these visual patterns. Figure 3 shows sample items for each of the four different types of word recognition tasks.

Because it is thought that phonological processing is, by its very nature, slower than orthographic processing (Waters and Seidenberg 1985; Seidenberg and McClelland 1989) and because it was expected that dyslexic subjects would recognize words more slowly than normal readers, the tasks were self-paced. Subjects were permitted to take as long as needed to process the information, but were encouraged to respond as quickly as possible. This subject-paced design insured that all subjects would spend most of their scanning time actually engaged in the sort of cognitive processing required by the tasks.

A fairly neutral baseline condition, which required each subject to visually fixate on a crosshair in the center of the monitor, was also performed. This control task provided visual input, but required no reading or linguistic processing and thus, when compared with the reading tasks, permitted the identification of the multiple language regions engaged by each of the four word recognition tasks. In addition, the phonological and orthographic versions of each task type—pronunciation and lexical decision making—were compared with each

	Pronunciation	Decision Making
Phonological	*Read aloud:*	*Which one sounds like a real word?*
	phalbap	jope - joak
	chirl	gaim - gome
Orthographic	*Read aloud:*	*Which one is a real word?*
	pharaoh	thurd - third
	choir	deep - deap

Figure 3.   Sample items for four word recognition tasks

other to identify regions with greater involvement in phonological and greater involvement in orthographic processing.

Normal word recognition: Controls were 14 men, ages 18 to 40, with no history of developmental disorder, who scored within an average or higher range on psychometric measures of reading and spelling upon direct examination at the time of study. This group performed all but the pseudoword pronunciation task with an average accuracy of greater than 90%. They read pseudowords with an average accuracy of 82%. In addition, the phonological tasks were performed more slowly than their orthographic counterparts, thus supporting the hypothesis that phonological processing is slower than is orthographic processing (Rumsey et al. 1997a).

Relative to the visual fixation condition, all four word recognition tasks elicited a left-lateralized stream of activation involving visual association regions in the lingual and fusiform gyri, perirolandic cortex (which contains sensory-motor regions for the hand and mouth), the thalamus and the anterior cingulate. Figure 4 illustrates these findings. Pronunciation and lexical decision making differed more in the patterns of activation elicited by them than did the phonological and orthographic versions of either pronunciation or lexical decision making. Both pronunciation tasks activated the left and right superior temporal gyri, with more extensive and intense activation seen on the left, but failed to activate the left inferior frontal region

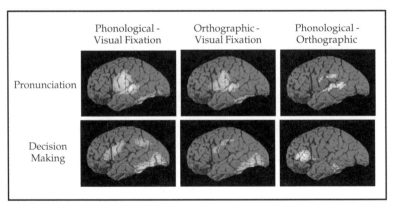

Figure 4. Regions in and near the cortex of the left hemisphere activated by control men (normal readers) during four word recognition tasks. Shown (in white) are regions activated by each task relative to the visual fixation control condition (left and center maps), as well as differences between the phonological and orthographic versions of the pronunciation and decision making tasks (on right). The phonological tasks were more activating than were their orthographic counterparts.

near Broca's area. Conversely, the lexical decision making tasks activated the left inferior cortex near Broca's area and bilateral parietal cortex, but failed to activate the superior temporal region.

Comparing the phonological and orthographic versions of each task type, the phonological versions were more activating of specific language regions than were their orthographic counterparts. The orthographic versions, in contrast, did not elicit greater activation than their phonological counterparts in other brain regions. The differences in activation appeared to be a matter of degree or intensity, rather than location. Thus, these results failed to provide evidence of "dual routes" subserving phonological and orthographic aspects of reading and were instead more compatible with single route models of word recognition.

In which regions were the phonological tasks more activating than the orthographic tasks? Phonological pronunciation (pseudoword reading) elicited greater activation of the left posterior superior temporal gyrus than did orthographic pronunciation (irregular word reading). Phonological decision making elicited greater activation of a left inferior frontal region (near and anterior to Broca's area). Thus, the pronunciation tasks identified posterior language regions where phonological processing was more activating than orthographic processing, and decision making identified anterior language regions where phonological processing was more activating.

Dyslexic word recognition: To determine the neural correlates of impaired word recognition and phonological processing in dyslexia, 17 dyslexic men were examined using PET and their scans were compared to those of the control men. The groups were well matched for age (18 to 40 years), handedness (all right-handed), socioeconomic status (all middle to upper), educational level (all at least high school diplomas and many with some college), and IQ (all at least average).

As expected, the dyslexic men performed each word recognition task more slowly and less accurately than their controls. Nonetheless, their average accuracy on the decision making tasks exceeded 80%. Their average accuracy for the pronunciation tasks was 62% for the real (irregularly spelled) words and 39% for the pseudowords. They were fully engaged in the tasks, even in those on which they performed poorly; and their pronunciations were generally partially correct, with errors confined to certain phonemes or sequences of phonemes. Like their controls, the dyslexic group found the phonological tasks more difficult than the orthographic tasks, as reflected in prolonged reaction times during phonological decision making as well as prolonged reaction times and reduced accuracy on phonological pronunciation.

Relative to the control group, the dyslexic group showed larger, more spatially extensive regions of activation and deactivation. This tendency was nonspecific, however, as it was distributed throughout the brain without significant differences in the intensity of the activations or in the levels of blood flow. These differences in spatial extent may well be an overall effect of the tasks being more difficult for the dyslexic men, as larger areas of activation have been noted to accompany lower levels of skill in some studies (Raichle et al. 1994).

As in controls, pronunciation activated the lingual and fusiform gyri, particularly on the left, the thalamic area, perirolandic cortex, and the anterior cingulate. The activations seen in the anterior cingulate, which are thought to be related to attention, were normal. Unusually large areas of deactivation encompassed significant portions of the inferior and middle temporal gyri and inferior parietal lobes bilaterally, the posterior midline parietal regions (paracentral, precuneus, posterior cingulate) and portions of bilateral prefrontal cortex.

As illustrated in figures 5 and 6, the major differences between the dyslexic and the control groups during pronunciation were localized to the temporal lobes, where dyslexics showed reduced blood flow. In contrast to the controls who activated the superior temporal gyrus bilaterally, but predominantly on the left, the dyslexic group showed reduced activation on the left and no activation on the right. These differences were greater during pseudoword than during real word reading. The reduced activation, together with the unusual deactivation seen in the dyslexic group, resulted in the differences during pronunciation being greater on the right than on the left.

During the decision making tasks, the dyslexic group activated bilateral lingual and fusiform gyri, particularly on the left, superior portions of the supramarginal gyri, the thalamic region, the left anterior cingulate, and the left inferior frontal region, as did controls. Both groups showed greater left inferior frontal and left anterior cingulate activation during phonological (relative to orthographic) decision making. (See figure 5.) The dyslexic group again showed extensive deactivation of the temporal lobes (relative to the visual fixation control). Relative to the controls, the dyslexic group showed lower blood flow in temporal cortex and inferior parietal cortex, particularly on the left, and particularly during phonological decision making due to their greater, more extensive deactivation of these regions and lesser activation of superior portions of inferior parietal cortex. (See figure 6.)

Thus, both during pronunciation tasks which activated the superior temporal gyri bilaterally and during decision making tasks which activated left inferior frontal language regions, the dyslexic group showed reduced blood flow in left and right temporal and parietal

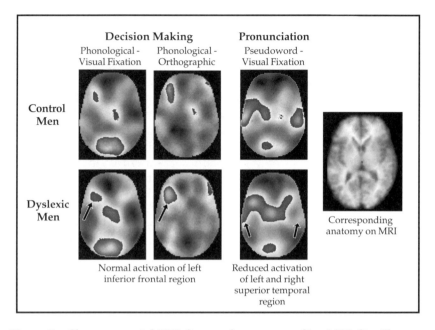

Figure 5.   Shown are axial PET slices and a corresponding MRI slice illustrating the normal activation of the left inferior frontal region elicited in dyslexic men by decision making, as well as their reduced activation of the left superior temporal region and lack of right superior temporal activation during pronunciation. Also illustrated is the tendency toward larger (more spatially extensive) areas of activation in the dyslexic men.

cortex. These differences resulted from the dyslexic group's reduced activation and increased deactivation of these regions relative to controls. In contrast, the dyslexic group showed normal activation of left inferior frontal cortex during decision making.

Consistent with the disproportionately greater phonological deficits seen in dyslexic men, group differences in blood flow were generally greater during the performance of the phonological tasks. However, the differences seen during the phonological, relative to the orthographic, tasks were primarily differences in magnitude, rather than in localization, again consistent with single route models of reading.

The localization of the differences seen across the word recognition tasks are generally consistent with the findings of the earlier auditory studies. Both examiner-paced auditory (nonreading) tasks and subject-paced visual word recognition tasks identified abnormalities in bilateral temporal and in left temporoparietal regions in men with developmental dyslexia. Both sets of findings are consistent with the hy-

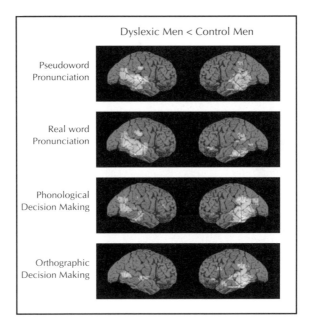

Figure 6. Shown are regions in and near the cortical surface of the left and right hemispheres in which task-related changes in blood flow, as measured with PET, differed in control and dyslexic men. The differences (mapped in white) represent regions of lower blood in dyslexic men relative to their controls. Some of these differences were due to reduced activation in dyslexic men; others, to greater deactivation.

pothesis that posterior portions of left hemisphere language networks, as well as homologous right-sided regions, are affected in dyslexia.

Relative to the orthographic tasks, the greater activation of both anterior and posterior language regions during the phonological tasks indicates that phonological processing cannot be localized to any single region of the brain. Rather, like many other neuropsychological constructs, this term encompasses a number of different subprocesses or cognitive operations. Along these lines, Wagner and Torgesen (1987) have discussed three different aspects of phonological processing with respect to reading: (1) phonological awareness, (2) phonological recoding to translate print into sound, and (3) phonetic recoding to maintain items in working memory. Deficits in phonological awareness (an early predictor of reading success) account substantially for word recognition deficits in dyslexia (Pennington et al. 1990). In contrast to this, deficits in verbal working memory may characterize only a subgroup of dyslexic adults (Pennington et al. 1990) and affect reading comprehension, rather than decoding. The good reading comprehension scores of the dyslexic men reported here suggest few deficits in verbal working memory in this group.

While the localization of these subcomponents requires further study, the findings reported here are consistent with their localization to different regions within a large scale language network. A phonological awareness task (auditory rhyme detection) elicited activation of left temporoparietal and superior temporal cortex in controls and decreased activation of these regions in dyslexic men (Rumsey et al. 1992). Given that phonological awareness is thought to be *causally* related to success in learning to read, the findings involving these regions may be causally related to dyslexia. Phonological recoding to translate print into sound was involved in the pronunciation tasks, which elicited activation of the left and right superior temporal gyri in controls and reduced activation of these regions in dyslexic men (Rumsey et al. 1997b). Finally, phonetic recoding to maintain items in working memory was involved in the lexical decision making tasks, particularly in the phonological version. Subjects used subvocal (silent) rehearsal to compare pronunciations in their minds. The left inferior frontal activation elicited by these tasks likely reflects the operation of this working memory component, as other work supports the involvement of this region in internal speech and verbal working memory (Bookheimer et al. 1995; McGuire et al. 1996; Paulesu et al. 1993).

The etiology of the differences in activation seen in posterior language regions in dyslexia is unknown, but may involve anatomic anomalies and/or genetic influences. Compelling evidence of a genetic etiology for dyslexia exists (DeFries and Alarcon 1996), and approximately two thirds of our sample reported a family history of reading problems. As described earlier, cortical anomalies, variably affecting left perisylvian regions, as well as right-sided cortex, may produce anomalous patterns of growth and connectivity, primarily affecting posterior language-related regions in dyslexic men (Galaburda et al. 1985). Studies in progress are examining anatomic MRI data collected on this sample, as well as functional relationships between brain regions thought to reflect connectivity.

AN fMRI STUDY OF VISUAL MOTION SENSITIVITY IN DYSLEXIA

Given neuropathological and neurophysiological evidence implicating the magnocellular pathways of the visual system discussed above, Eden et al. (1996) designed an fMRI study to examine the integrity of this system in dyslexia. A subgroup of the PET sample described above, consisting of six dyslexic men and six controls, and two new controls participated in this study.

To test the hypothesis of a selective magnocellular visual processing deficit in dyslexia, sensitivity to visual motion was evaluated both behaviorally and physiologically. To evaluate motion sensitivity using psychophysical testing, subjects were presented with successive one-second presentations of a low contrast (minimal difference in grayness between dark dots and a lighter background) display of moving dots differing only in their velocity and asked to judge whether the velocity of a second stimulus was slower or faster than that of a target stimulus. Relative to their controls, the dyslexics judged the velocities less accurately.

To determine their underlying physiological sensitivity to motion, fMRI scans were obtained while subjects visually fixated on a central crosshair during three conditions: (1) a control condition in which the central crosshair was presented on an isoluminant background (2) a *pattern* condition, in which subjects viewed a stationary, high-contrast black and white pattern, and finally (3) a *motion* condition, in which they viewed a low contrast random field of moving dots. To identify regions activated by visual pattern and visual motion, the latter conditions each were compared to the common baseline, the visual fixation control.

As expected, all subjects exhibited similar responses to the pattern stimulus, which activated primary and secondary visual association areas (V1/V2) in posterior occipital cortex and extrastriate visual areas (inferior temporal/fusiform gyrus). Thus, the dyslexic subjects demonstrated a normal response to pattern with activation of the above-mentioned occipital and inferior temporal regions, providing evidence of the integrity of the pattern/form visual system thought to be dominated by parvocellular input. In contrast to this, the physiological responses of the dyslexics to visual motion differed dramatically from those of controls. Visual motion elicited activation in the visual motion area V5/MT bilaterally in each control subject, confirming prior demonstrations of robust motion sensitivity in this region in normal subjects (Watson et al. 1993). In contrast, of the six dyslexic men examined, only one showed detectable activation within this region (as identified by Watson et al. 1993), and this subject activated V5/MT only on the left side of the brain. Results for the control and dyslexic groups (averaged across individuals) are illustrated in figure 7.

Interestingly, responses were seen in other motion sensitive visual cortical areas in the anterior temporal and parietal lobes in both groups. The preserved function of these additional motion sensitive areas in dyslexia requires further investigation, but one could speculate that the failure to activate V5/MT and accompanying behavioral deficits might result from disrupted interaction of these multiple mo-

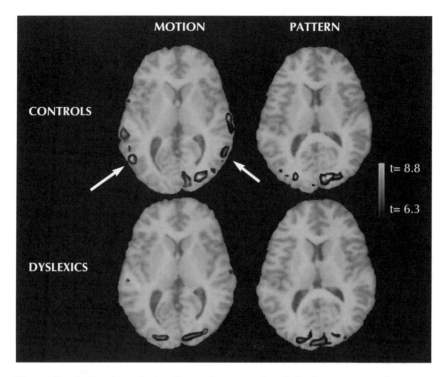

Figure 7. Activation of visual areas by control and dyslexic men as shown on axial fMRI slices. Dyslexic men activated V1/V2 in response to pattern, but failed to activate MT/V5 in response to visual motion. Arrows (near brain at upper left) indicate the activation of MT/V5 in control men.

tion processing areas that probably rely on exquisite temporal synchronization. Also, disruption of V5/MT activity may be expected to interfere with re-entrant signals to other visual cortical areas as well as to the oculomotor apparatus. This may provide an explanation for eye movement abnormalities observed in some dyslexics (Eden et al. 1994). Such abnormalities have been proposed as an explanation for reading impairment, but may in fact be a reflection of inaccurate magnocellular processing, one of a constellation of neuronal abnormalities in dyslexia. Visual system abnormalities may be one component, possibly a biological marker, for a complex disorder that involves numerous components, including the well-established deficit in phonological awareness.

SUMMARY AND FUTURE DIRECTIONS

This chapter has described the first PET and fMRI studies of regional cerebral blood flow in dyslexia, studies which have investigated both language-based and visually-based abnormalities in men with clear, persisting cases of dyslexia. Results of both sets of studies suggest bilateral reductions in task-related activation in posterior temporal brain regions and nearby inferior parietal and occipital brain regions. Both the language studies and visual studies have identified significant neural correlates of the behavioral deficits associated with dyslexia. PET studies of word recognition have implicated posterior language regions, including left and right temporal and left inferior parietal regions, in dyslexia with preservation of more anterior language regions in the left inferior frontal lobe. An fMRI study of visual motion processing has implicated dysfunction of the transient, magnocellular visual pathway in dyslexia with preservation of visual association regions subserving pattern processing, thought to reflect the function of the sustained, parvocellular pathway. Studies in progress are exploring relationships between the above findings and potential subtle alterations in the neuroanatomy of these regions and/or altered functional connectivity of these regions. Relationships between physiological abnormalities and behavioral variables, such as the severity of dyslexia, are also underway to further characterize the nature of some of the differences seen.

Whether and how word recognition deficits and visual processing abnormalities, both accompanied by reduced activation in and near posterior temporal brain regions, are related remains an open question in need of further study. One possibility is that some common underlying deficit in the transient, or rapid, processing of temporal information contributes to both categories of deficit. Combining the experimental results from neuroimaging studies of reading and reading-related processing with those demonstrating a magnocellular visual system deficit, the superior temporal/inferior parietal areas emerge as likely candidates for the principal locus of cerebral dysfunction in dyslexia. Visual input to the temporoparietal area is predominantly provided by the magnocellular system. This originates in the magnocellular layers of the lateral geniculate nucleus (LGN) and projects to area MT/V5 (Tootell and Taylor 1995) and to parietal cortex bilaterally (Livingstone and Hubel 1988; Maunsell and Newsome 1987; Ungerleider and Mishkin 1982; Van Essen and Maunsell 1983). Functional neuroimaging studies have confirmed responses to visual motion processing in area V5/MT of the human visual system, together with increased activity in inferior parietal areas (Eden et al. 1996). Similarly, PET studies examining reading-related processes have identified the superior/middle temporal gyri and, less consistently, the inferior parietal lobe to be active (Bookheimer et al. 1995; Rumsey et al. 1997a, b). Also, it appears that in comparison to some of the frontal areas that have been associated with increased blood flow during functional imaging studies of language, these posterior areas are more actively engaged during pronunciation (Bookheimer et al. 1995; Rumsey et al. 1997b).

Functional magnetic resonance imaging now offers unprecedented opportunities for imaging brain function in children and for understanding the variability associated with developmental reading disorders. Whether the findings reported above will generalize to other samples, particularly those with less widely accepted diagnoses due to low IQs or less stable diagnoses, that is, of individuals with more transient reading difficulties, is an empirical question. Studies of dyslexic children and of related reading disorders will doubtlessly shed light on the nature of the multiple deficits associated with poor reading, their interrelationships, and the causative versus correlational nature of their associations with dyslexia.

ACKNOWLEDGMENT

The authors wish to thank Brian C. Donohue for his helpful review of this manuscript and for his assistance with the figures.

REFERENCES

American Psychiatric Association 1994. *Diagnostic and Statistical Manual of Mental Disorders* (4th ed.). Washington, D.C.

Andreasen, N. C., Flaum, M., Swayze II, V., O'Leary, D. S., Alliger, R., Cohen, G., Ehrhardt, J., and Yuh, W. T. 1993. Intelligence and brain structure in normal individuals. *American Journal of Psychiatry* 150:130–34.

Bishop, D. V. M., and Adams, C. 1990. A prospective study of the relationship between specific language impairment, phonological disorders and reading retardation. *Journal of Child Psychology and Psychiatry* 31:1027–50.

Blachman, B. A. 1991. Getting ready to read. In *The Language Continuum: From Infancy to Literacy*, ed. J. F. Kavanagh. Parkton, MD: York Press.

Bookheimer, S. Y., Zeffiro, T. A., Blaxton, T., Gaillard, W., and Theodore, W. 1995. Regional cerebral blood flow during object naming and word reading. *Human Brain Mapping* 3:93–106.

Bowers, P. G., and Wolf, M. 1993. Theoretical links among naming speed, precise timing mechanisms and orthographic skill in dyslexia. *Reading & Writing* 5:69–85.

Bradley, L., and Bryant, P. E. 1983. Categorizing sounds and learning to read: A causal connection. *Nature* 301:419–21.

Brady, S. 1986. Short-term memory, phonological processing and reading ability. *Annals of Dyslexia* 36:138–53.

Brady, S. A., and Shankweiler, D. 1991. *Phonological Processing in Literacy: A Tribute to Isabelle Y. Liberman*. Hillsdale, New Jersey: Lawrence Erlbaum Associates.

Breitmeyer, B. G. 1980. Unmasking visual masking: A look at the "why: behind the veil of how." *Psychological Review* 87:52–69.

Coltheart, M., Curtis, B., Atkins, P., and Haller, M. 1993. Models of reading aloud: Dual-route and parallel-distributed processing approaches. *Psychological Review* 100:589–608.

Conners, F., and Olson, R. 1990. Reading comprehension in dyslexic and normal readers: a component skills analysis. In *Comprehension Processes in Reading*, eds. D. A. Balota, G. B. Flores d'Arcais, and K. Rayner. Hillsdale, NJ: Lawrence Erlbaum Associates.

Corbetta, M., Miezin, F. M., Dobmeyer, S., Shulman, G. L., and Petersen, S. E. 1990. Attentional modulation of neural processing of shape, color, and velocity in humans. *Science* 248:1556–59.

DeFries, J. C., and Alarcon, M. 1996. Genetics of specific reading disability. *Mental Retardation and Developmental Disabilities* 2:39–47.

Eden, G. F., Stein, J. F., Wood, H. M., and Wood, F. B. 1994. Differences in eye movements and reading problems in dyslexic and normal children. *Vision Research* 34:1345–58.

Eden, G. F., VanMeter, J. W., Rumsey, J. M., Maisog, J. M., Woods, R. P., and Zeffiro, T. A. 1996. Abnormal processing of visual motion in dyslexia revealed by functional brain imaging. *Nature* 382: 66–69.

Eden, G., and Zeffiro, T. 1996. PET and fMRI in the detection of task related brain activity: Implications for the study of brain development. In *Developmental Neuroimaging: Mapping the Development of Brain and Behavior*, eds. R. W. Thatcher, G. R. Lyon, J. Rumsey, and N. Krasnegor. San Diego:Academic Press, Inc.

Ehri, L. C., and Wilce, L. S. 1985. Movement into reading: Is the first stage of printed word learning visual or phonetic? *Reading Research Quarterly* 20:163–79.

Friedman, R. F., Ween, J. E., and Albert, M. L. 1993. Alexia. In *Clinical Neuropsychology*, eds. K. M. Heilman and E. Valenstein. New York: Oxford University Press.

Galaburda, A. M., Sherman, G. F., Rosen, G. D., Aboitiz, F., and Geschwind, N. 1985. Developmental dyslexia: four consecutive patients with cortical anomalies. *Annals of Neurology* 18:222–33.

Goswami, U. 1986. Children's use of analogy in learning to read: A developmental study. *Journal of Experimental Child Psychology* 42:73–83.

Henderson, V. W. 1986. Anatomy of posterior pathways in reading: A reassessment. *Brain and Language* 29:119–33.

Kaplan, E., and Shapley, R. M. 1982. X and Y cells in the lateral geniculate nucleus of macaque monkeys. *Journal of Physiology* 330:125–43.

Knopman, D. S., Rubens, A. B., Klassen, A. C., and Meyer, M. W. 1982. Regional cerebral blood flow correlates of auditory processing. *Archives of Neurology* 39:487–93.

Krasuski, J., Horwitz, B., and Rumsey, J. M. 1996. A survey of functional and anatomical neuroimaging techniques. In *Neuroimaging: A Window to the*

Neurological Foundations of Learning and Behavior in Children, eds. G. R. Lyon and J. M. Rumsey. Baltimore: Brookes.

Liberman, I. Y., and Shankweiler, D. 1985. Phonology and the problems of learning to read and write. *Remedial and Special Education* 6:8–17.

Livingstone, M., and Hubel, D. 1988. Segregation of form, colour, movement and depth: Anatomy, physiology, and perception. *Science* 240:740–49.

Livingstone, M. S., Rosen, G. D., Drislane, F. W., and Galaburda, A. M. 1991. Physiological and natomical evidence for a magnocellular deficit in developmental dyslexia. *Proceedings of the National Academy of Science* 88:7943–47.

Lovegrove, W. 1993. Weakness in transient visual system: A causal factor in dyslexia? *Annals of the New York Academy of Sciences* 14:57–69.

Lovegrove, W., and Brown, C. 1978. Development of information processing in normal and disabled readers. *Journal of Perceptual and Motor Skills* 46:1047–54.

Lovegrove, W. J., Heddle, M., and Slaghuis, W. 1980. Reading disability: Spatial frequency specific deficits in visual information store. *Neuropsychologia* 18:111–15.

Mann, V. A., and Brady, S. 1988. Reading disability: The role of language deficiencies. *Journal of Consulting and Clinical Psychology* 56:811–16.

Martin, F., and Lovegrove, W. 1984. The effect of field size and luminance on contrast sensitivity differences between specifically reading disabled and normal children. *Neuropsychologia* 22:73–77.

Martin, F., and Lovegrove, W. 1988. Uniform and field flicker in control and specifically-disabled readers. *Perception* 17:203–14.

Maunsell, J. H. R., and Newsome, W. T. 1987. Visual processing in monkey extrastriate cortex. *Annual Review of Neuroscience*, 10:363–401.

Mazziotta, J. C., Phelps, M. E., Carson, R. E., and Kuhl, D. E. 1982. Tomographic mapping of human cerebral metabolism: Auditory stimulation. *Neurology* 2:921–37.

McCarthy, R. A., and Warrington, E. K. 1990. *Cognitive Neuropsychology: A Clinical Introduction*. San Diego: Academic Press, Inc.

McGuire, P. K., Silbersweig, D. A., Murray, R. M., David, A. S., Frackowiak, R. S., and Frith, C. D. 1996. Functional anatomy of inner speech and auditory verbal imagery. *Psychological Medicine* 26:29–38.

Mesulam M. M. 1990. Large scale neurocognitive networks and distributed processing for attention, language and memory. *Annals of Neurology* 28:587–613.

Nobre, A. C., Allison, T., and McCarthy, G. 1994. Word recognition in the human temporal lobe. *Nature* 372:260–63.

Olson, R., Forsberg, H., Wise, B., and Rack, J. 1994. Measurement of word recognition, orthographic, and phonological skills. In *Frames of Reference for the Assessment of Learning Disabilities*, ed. G. R. Lyon. Baltimore: Brookes.

Olson, R. K., Wise, B., Conners, F., Rack, J., and Fulker, D. 1989. Specific deficits in component reading and language skills: Genetic and environmental influences. *Journal of Learning Disabilities* 22:239–348.

Paulesu, E., Frith, C. D., and Frackowiak, R. S. J. 1993. The neural correlates of the verbal component of working memory. *Nature* 362:334–42.

Pennington, B. F., Lefly, D. L., Van Orden, G. C., Bookman, O. M., and Smith, S. D. 1987. Is phonology bypassed in normal or dyslexic development? *Annals of Dyslexia* 37:62–89.

Pennington, B. F., Van Orden, G. C., Smith, S. D., Green, P. A., and Haith, M. M. 1990. Phonological processing skills and deficits in adult dyslexics. *Child Development* 61:1753–78.

Petersen, S. E., Fox, P. T., Posner, M. I., Mintun, M., and Raichle, M. E. 1989. Positron emission tomographic studies of the processing of single words. *Journal of Cognitive Neuroscience* 1:153–70.

Petersen, S. E., Fox, P. T., Snyder, A. Z., and Raichle, M. E. 1990. Activation of extrastriate and frontal cortical areas by visual words and word-like stimuli. *Science* 249:1041–44.

Plaut, D. C., McClelland, J. L., Seidenberg, M. S., and Patterson, K. 1996. Understanding normal and impaired word reading: Computational principles in quasi-regular domains. *Psychological Review* 103:56–115.

Raichle, M. E., Fiez, J. A., Videen, T. O., MacLeod, A. M., Pardo, J. V., Fox P. T., and Petersen, S. E. 1994. Practice-related changes in human brain functional anatomy during nonmotor learning. *Cerebral Cortex* 4:8–26.

Rumsey, J. M., Andreason, P., Zametkin, A. J., Aquino, T., King, A. C., Hamburger, S. D., Pikus, A., Rapoport, J. L., and Cohen, R. M. 1992. Failure to activate the left temporoparietal cortex in dyslexia: An oxygen 15 positron emission tomographic study. *Archives of Neurology* 49:527–34.

Rumsey, J. M., Andreason, P., Zametkin, A. J., King, A. C., Hamburger, S. D., Aquino, T., Hanahan, A. P., Pikus, A., and Cohen, R. M. 1994a. Right frontotemporal activation by tonal memory in dyslexia, an O-15 PET study. *Biological Psychiatry* 36: 171–80.

Rumsey, J. M., Horwitz, B., Donohue, B. C., Nace, K., Maisog, J. M., and Andreason, P. 1997a. Phonologic and orthographic components of word recognition: A PET-rCBF study. *Brain* 120:739–60.

Rumsey, J. M., Nace, K., Donohue, B. C., Wise, D., Maisog, J. M., and Andreason, P. 1997b. A positron emission tomographic study of impaired word recognition and phonological processing in dyslexic men. *Archives of Neurology* 54:562–73.

Rumsey, J. M., Zametkin, A. J., Andreason, P., Hanahan, A. P., Hamburger, S. D., Aquino, T., King, A. C., Pikus, A., and Cohen, R. M. 1994b. Normal activation of frontotemporal language cortex in dyslexia, as measured with oxygen 15 positron emission tomography. *Archives of Neurology* 51:27–38.

Satz, P., and Morris, R. 1981. Learning disability subtypes: A review. In *Neuropsychological and Cognitive Processes in Reading*, eds. F. J. Pirozzolo and M. C. Wittrock. New York: Academic Press.

Schiller, P. H., and Colby, C. L. 1983. The responses of single cells in the lateral geniculate nucleus of the rhesus monkey to color and luminance contrast. *Vision Research*, 23:1631–41.

Seidenberg, M. S., and McClelland, J. L. 1989. A distributed developmental model of word recognition and naming. *Psychological Review* 96: 523–68.

Shaywitz, S. E., Shaywitz, B. A., Fletcher, J. M., and Escobar, M. D. 1990. Prevalence of reading disability in boys and girls. Results of the Connecticut Longitudinal Study. *Journal of the American Medical Association* 264:998–1002.

Siegel, L. S. 1992. An evaluation of the discrepancy definition of dyslexia. *Journal of Learning Disabilities* 25:618–29.

Stanley, G., Smith, G. A., and Howell, G. A. 1983. Eye movements and sequential tracking in dyslexic and control children. *British Journal of Psychology* 74: 181–87.

Stanovich, K. E., and Siegel, L. S. 1994. Phenotypic performance profile of children with reading disabilities: A regression-based test of the phonological-core variable-difference model. *Journal of Educational Psychology* 86:24–53.

Studdert-Kennedy, M., and Mody, M. 1995. Auditory temporal perception deficits in the reading-impaired: A critical review of the evidence. *Psychonomic Bulletin and Review* 1:508–14.

Tallal, P., Miller, S., and Fitch, R. H. 1993. Neurobiological basis of the case for the preeminence of temporal processing. In *Temporal Information Processing in the Nervous System: Special Reference to Dyslexia and Dysphasia*, eds. P. Tallal, A. M. Galaburda, and R. R. Llinás. New York: The New York Academy of Sciences.

Tootell, R. B., Reppas, J. B., Kwong, K. K., Malach, R., Born, R. T., Brady, T. J., Rosen, B. R., and Belliveau, J. W. 1995. Functional analysis of human MT and related visual cortical areas using magnetic resonance imaging. *Journal of Neuroscience* 15:3215–30.

Tootell, R. B., and Taylor, J. B. 1995. Anatomical evidence for MT and additional cortical visual areas in humans. *Cerebral Cortex* 5:39–55.

Ungerleider, L. G., and Mishkin, M. 1982. Two cortical visual systems. In *Analysis of Visual Behavior*, eds. D. J. Ingle, M. A. Goodale, and R. J. W. Mansfield. Cambridge: MIT Press.

Van Essen, D., and Maunsell, J. H. R. 1983. Hierarchical organization and functional streams in the visual cortex. *Trends in Neurosciences* 9:370–75.

Vellutino, F., Scanlon, D. M., and Chen, D. S. 1995. The increasingly inextricable relationship between orthographic and phonological coding in learning to read: Some reservations about current methods of operationalizing orthographic coding. In *The Varieties of Orthographic Knowledge II: Relationships to Phonology, Reading and Writing*, ed. V. W. Berninger. Dordrecht, Netherlands: Kluwer Academic Publishers.

Wagner, R. K., and Torgeson, J. K. 1987. The nature of phonological processing and its causal role in the acquisition of reading skills. *Psychological Bulletin* 101:193–212.

Walsh, V. 1995. Reading between the laminae. *Current Biology* 5:1216–17.

Waters, G. S., and Seidenberg, M. S. 1985. Spelling-sound effects in reading: Time-course and decision criteria. *Brain and Cognition* 13:557–72.

Watson, J. D. G., Myers, R., Frackowiak, R. S. J., Hajnal, J. V., Woods, R. P., Mazziotta, J. C., Shipp, S., and Zeki, S. 1993. Area V5 of the human brain: Evidence from a combined study using positron emission tomography and magnetic resonance imaging. *Cerebral Cortex* 3:79–94.

Wiederholt, J. L., and Bryant, B. R. 1992. *Gray Oral Reading Tests, Third edition*. Austin, TX: PRO-ED.

Willows, D. M. 1991. Visual processes in learning disabilities. In *Learning About Learning Disabilities*, ed. B. Y. L. Wong. San Diego, CA: Academic Press.

Chapter • 4

Genetics of Reading Disability
Further Evidence for a Gene on Chromosome 6

S. D. Smith,
A. M. Brower,
L. R. Cardon, and
J. C. DeFries

Several different types of studies have indicated that specific reading disability is influenced by genetic factors. Twin studies have shown that a substantial portion of the variation in reading ability can be attributed to genes (DeFries et al. 1993), and segregation analysis of family data has shown that a few major genes may be involved (Pennington et al. 1991; Gilger et al. 1994). Discovery of such genes would allow the identification of children at higher risk for reading disability, and determination of the function of the genes would reveal important biological factors involved in the reading process. Identification of the genes that underlie complex behavioral processes is difficult, however, and the necessary molecular laboratory techniques and statistical analysis methods are still evolving.

The most commonly used method of gene identification depends upon the phenomenon of gene linkage. Genes are arrayed in linear fashion along chromosomes, the packaged lengths of DNA contained in the nucleus of each cell. There are 23 pairs of chromosomes in all, with one member of each pair inherited from each parent. Similarly, one chromosome from each pair is selected at random for inclusion in the egg or the sperm for transmission to the next generation. Since the transmission of genes is done through the chromosomes, genes that are located close together on the same chromosome tend to be transmitted together and are said to be linked. Genes may have alternate forms, called alleles, that differ in their genetic code; for example, in a gene that influences eye color, one allele may code for blue and the other may code for brown. Allelic differences allow a particular chromosomal region to be followed as it is transmitted through a family. For example, if a person has a blue allele on the chromosome he inherited from his father and a brown allele on the chromosome from his mother, it can be determined which of the two chromosomes was transmitted to his child by looking at the eye color allele that he or she inherited. This gene "marks" that particular part of the chromosome so that it can be followed through the family. Now let us postulate that this father's paternal side has another gene for hand development which has two alleles, a normal allele and one that produces polydactyly (an extra finger). Further, let us suppose that everyone in the family who inherited the blue allele also had polydactyly, and no one with the brown allele inherited polydactyly. This would indicate that the eye color gene and the polydactyly gene were linked on the same chromosome, so that both were inherited together. Thus, by knowing where the eye color gene is located on the chromosome, one can learn where the polydactyly gene is located. If one wants to find out where a gene for a genetic condition is located, then, the transmission of that gene can be compared to the transmission of many different "marker" genes with known locations on the chromosomes, to see if any of these marker genes are linked to the gene for that condition. The statistical analysis to determine if the marker and the condition are really inherited together, more than would be expected by coincidence, is called linkage analysis. In practice, alleles that represent variable regions of DNA code are used as markers, since the alleles can be detected more easily and more reliably than gene variations. If linkage analysis finds that a set of marker alleles (representing a region of a specific chromosome being inherited through a family) is found significantly more often in family members with reading disability, for example, this would indicate that a gene included in that region influences reading.

Several methods of linkage analysis are available for detection of genes with major influences on a condition, and now there are also methods for detection of genes with more subtle influences. The development of the molecular DNA markers which have many alleles and are closely spaced along the chromosomes has made it possible to examine all of the chromosomes for linkage, so that, if a gene exists that has an influence on a condition, it can be found. However, the ability of linkage analysis to detect the linkage is also dependent upon the correct analysis technique and the appropriate sample of families.

The most commonly used linkage analysis methods can be classified into "parametric" and "nonparametric" types. In parametric linkage analysis, entire families are studied, and parameters specifying the frequency of the gene and the way it is inherited (dominant or recessive, for example) are used to give the most accurate information on the location of the gene and its distance from the marker genes. The diagnosis is specified for each family member in the analysis, and the presence or absence of the condition is compared with each person's marker alleles to see if they are transmitted together. This type of linkage analysis has been used for the localization of genes for many genetic diseases, such as cystic fibrosis, muscular dystrophy, and Huntington's disease.

For complex traits such as reading disability, where the mode of inheritance of a specific gene is not known, a nonparametric linkage analysis technique is most likely to give accurate results. In these methods, limited sets of relatives (usually pairs of siblings, but sometimes other sets of 2 or 3 relatives) are compared to see if individuals with the genetic condition share the same marker alleles. These allele sharing methods are based on the assumption that individuals in a family who are alike for the genetic condition will also be alike for the linked alleles. This method is accurate as long as the shared alleles are "identical by descent," meaning that they were inherited from the same common ancestor. To use the example above, this would mean that two siblings who share the polydactyly trait should also share the blue-eyed allele. However, this could easily happen by coincidence if the polydactyly gene and the eye-color gene were on separate chromosomes, but both parents had a blue allele, and one child inherited the allele from the mother and the other child inherited it from the father. In this case, the blue alleles in the siblings are not "identical by descent," and the fact that they share both polydactyly and eye color does not indicate linkage. Nonparametric analysis does not require any assumptions about the mode of inheritance or other parameters, but is somewhat limited since the assumption of identity by descent of the shared alleles is not always proven unless both parents are also typed for the marker alleles. Since the presence or absence of the genetic condition does not have to be specified in the parents, this type of analysis is also advantageous with a condition in which diagnosis is difficult with certain age groups, or if the gene for the condition shows decreased penetrance (that is, someone can have the gene for the condition, but not actually have the condition itself). For example, diagnosis of reading disability may be difficult in adults who have compensated for earlier reading problems; they may have the gene influencing reading disability, but their reading level would be adequate.

Previous work by our group utilized nonparametric analysis to identify a region of the short arm of chromosome 6 (referred to as 6p) as highly likely to contain a gene influencing reading disability. Using a sample of 46 dyzygotic twin pairs in which at least one twin had reading disability, nonparametric linkage analysis using methods developed by Cardon and Fulker (1994) indicated linkage with a significance level of 0.009 for the interval between two DNA markers, D6S105 and TNFB (Cardon et al. 1994, 1995). These markers represent alterations in DNA sequence which do not have a known genetic or phenotypic effect, but merely mark positions along the chromosome and can be used to localize other genes. Thus, these results suggested that there is a gene between these two markers which has an influence on reading disability. Similar analyses in an independent set of families have confirmed the localization to this region (Grigorenko et al. 1997), covering about a 10–16 cM region. We have expanded our twin sample from 46 to 176 sibling pairs, and are examining additional markers in the region to refine the linkage. This chapter presents a preliminary analysis of the genotyping that has been completed to date.

Association analysis can be an additional method for detection of linkage. When two genes are linked within a family, specific alleles for both genes will be inherited together because they are close together on the same parental chromosomes. Between families, however, the specific alleles that are linked should be different. For example, in one family an allele causing a genetic disorder may be linked to allele #1 of a marker; but in another family, the causal allele could be linked to allele #2 of the same marker; and in still another family it could be linked to allele #3. The important point in linkage is that the two linked genes are transmitted together from generation to generation, regardless of the particular alleles coded for in those genes. On the other hand, association refers to the situation when a particular allele of one gene is found more often in individuals (not relatives) who have a particular allele of another gene. The most notable associations have been between alleles producing certain HLA types and alleles producing some genetic diseases. This type of association explains the observation that certain subtypes of HLA—DR and DQ—are found more often in individuals with insulin dependent diabetes mellitus than in individuals who are not diabetic.

Association can reflect several situations. The associated marker allele may be very closely linked to the allele influencing the disorder, resulting in linkage disequilibrium. Given that the mutation influencing the disorder occurred on a specific ancestral chromosome, alleles at loci that were tightly linked on that chromosome will stay with it through a number of generations until there has been enough random recombination to separate them. Thus, the persistence of association through linkage disequilibrium is dependent upon the distance between the loci and the number of generations since the mutation. If association is caused by linkage disequilibrium, the marker locus should show both linkage and association.

Association analysis is often done by comparing the marker alleles in a population with a genetic condition with the marker alleles in a separate control population without the condition. This can produce spurious linkage if the two populations are not sampled from the same overall population; for example, if they are from different ethnic groups (Kidd 1993). If the population with the condition is from one ethnic group, and the control population is from a different ethnic group, a marker allele may be found more often in the group with the condition only because the marker allele happens to be more frequent in that ethnic group. This problem can be avoided if the controls are taken from within the same family. In the Transmission Disequilibrium Test, the control alleles are the alleles that are not transmitted by a parent to a child with the genetic condition. If the marker gene that was transmitted to the affected children carries a specific allele significantly more often than the non-transmitted gene, it is evidence of linkage and association between the gene for the condition and the marker allele.

The most serious problem with using association analysis to detect linkage is that it requires that individuals with the condition share a common ancestor. In a heterogeneous population where the allele producing the condition could have arisen in a number of independent ancestors with different alleles at the marker gene, significant association with one marker allele will not be seen.

A TWIN STUDY

The Learning Disabilities Research Center project directed by Dr. J. C. DeFries at the University of Colorado has been ascertaining a large series of identical and fraternal twins for genetic analysis. At least one twin in each pair was reported by his or her teacher to have a reading disability, and a battery of reading and spelling tests was given to confirm this. These tests included the Peabody Individual Achievement Tests and the Wechsler Intelligence Scale for Children-Revised or the Wechsler Adult Intelligence Scale-Revised. A quantitative measure of reading ability was obtained for each subject by deriving a discriminant score from the PIAT Reading Recognition, Reading Comprehension, and Spelling subtests, based on a function previously shown by DeFries and colleagues to differentiate good and poor readers (DeFries, Fulker, and LaBuda 1987). All twins had a verbal or full scale IQ score of at least 90, and no other known neurological or sensory handicaps that could account for the reading disability.

Following informed consent, blood samples were obtained from the participants in this study as follows. Monozygotic (identical) twin pairs were not sampled except if a non-twin sibling was also tested and sampled. All consenting dyzygotic twins were sampled, along with available non-twin siblings, and blood samples were also requested from both biological parents. In some cases, grandparents were also sampled, which helped determine the identity by descent of the marker alleles.

DNA was extracted from the white blood cells in the samples, and specific marker sections of the DNA were amplified by the PCR (polymerase chain reaction) technique. With this procedure, a small piece of marker DNA is defined by known primer sequences at the beginning and the end of the piece, and many copies are made of the piece between the primers. This amplification gives enough copies of the piece of DNA for analysis. These markers contain short codes of DNA that are repeated a given number of times, and the number of repeats constitutes the difference between alleles for a marker. Thus, the different alleles are defined as differences in the length of the piece of DNA; one allele will have a smaller number of repeats and be shorter in length, while another allele will have more repeats and be longer in length. With some markers, there can be many different allele sizes.

Because our previous results suggested a gene in the region of D6S105, a marker on the short arm of chromosome 6, a series of DNA markers were typed that were known to be in this same region. Most of these markers were developed and mapped by Genethon, and their positions and distances along the chromosome are available on the Internet at http://www.genethon.fr/ or through the Genome Data Base at http://gdbwww.gdb.org/. Genotyping was done under the direction of Dr. Cardon at Sequana, Inc. using an ABI 377 DNA sequencer for genotyping. D6S105 is now considered to be equivalent to another marker named D6S464, and the current order and distances between the markers are given in figure 1. It should be noted that refinements in this information are being made continually, and the current order is different from previously used orders in our own work and in that by Grigorenko et al. (1997).

For this preliminary analysis, the sibhe program of the GAS (Genetic Analysis System) version 2.0 was used (©A. Young, Oxford University, 1993–1995). This program implements the Haseman-Elston method of sib pair analysis (Haseman and Elston 1972), which also formed the basis of the Cardon and Fulker linkage method used previously. In the Haseman-Elston method, the proportion of alleles at a marker that is identical by descent (IBD) in a pair of siblings is regressed against their phenotypic similarity, as measured by the square of the difference in their discriminant scores. Full siblings and dyzy-gotic twins will share 0, 1, or 2 alleles identical by descent at each marker. The more similar the siblings are in phenotype (that is, the smaller the difference in scores), the more alike the siblings should also be in genotype; they should inherit the same genes from their parents and have a higher IBD score. Linkage is accepted if the slope of the regression line is negative and is significantly different from 0. To test whether the gene is more likely to be present in more severely affected individuals, linkage analysis was done first with all of the sibling pairs; and then the population was limited to pairs in which at least one sibling had a discriminant score of less than –0.75; then to those pairs in which at least one had a score of less than –1.0; and finally to those in which at least one had a score of less than –1.5.

Association analysis was done using the asstdt program of the GAS package, which implements the Transmission Disequilibrium Test method of Spielman et al. (1993). Since the sample of affected individuals needs to be independent, if more than one sibling was included in the analysis, the information from each sibling group was averaged. In the initial analysis, only those siblings who had a discriminant score of less than –0.5 were included. Subsequently, the population was restricted further to those in which the discriminant score was less than –1.0.

The markers from chromosome 6p21.3 and their respective significance levels are shown in table I. From these data, increasing significance was seen for markers D6S105 and D6S258 as the population was restricted to include more severely affected subjects, although this tended to plateau when the selection went beyond a discriminant score less than –1.0. This could mean that the sample was not further enriched for the putative reading disability gene beyond that point,

Table I. Sib pair linkage analysis between reading disability and chromosome 6p21.3 markers

Discriminant score selection				
Marker	All $n = 176$	≤ 0.75 $n = 112$	≤ 1.0 $n = 91$	≤ 1.5 $n = 51$
D6S461	0.57	0.48	0.43	0.36
D6S306	0.49	0.28	0.25	0.072
D6S105/464	0.18	0.064	**0.046**	**0.03**
D6S258	0.064	**0.023**	**0.015**	**0.024**
D6S276	0.79	0.69	0.68	0.57
D6S439	0.32	0.19	0.19	0.24
D6S291	0.82	0.77	0.70	0.87
D6S1011	0.37	0.54	0.41	0.47
D6S1019	0.44	0.31	0.27	0.39

but the results could also reflect the decreasing sample size. As shown in figure 1, the two markers that showed p values less than 0.05 are thought to be quite close together; and the results for D6S306, the other marker in that group, began to approach significance as the population was restricted further. The remaining markers showed no evidence of linkage.

These results are shown graphically in figure 2. For clarity, only the results of the entire population and the population restricted to at least one sibling with a discriminant score of less than –1.0 are shown. This graph adds the information from a previously typed marker, TNFB (now known as LTA), which is located between the three clustered genes and D6S276. GAS sibhe analysis of the genotypes from that marker gave a p value of 0.12 for the entire sample, and 0.077 for the population restricted to at least one sibling with a discriminant score of less than –1.0.

Using the Transmission Disequilibrium Test as implemented by the asstdt program in the GAS package, significant association was found for one allele, #6 of the marker D6S306. In the initial analysis with all siblings having a discriminant score of less than –0.5, a p value of 0.037 was obtained for that allele. When the population was restricted to those with a discriminant score of less than –1.0, the p value for the same allele of D6S306 became 0.042.

A READING GENE

The results of the GAS sib pair analysis of the expanded data set is consistent with our previous results demonstrating localization of a gene influencing reading disability to chromosome 6p21.3, and helps narrow the region containing the gene to a linkage group containing 3 markers, D6S306, D6S105/646, and D6S258. As in our previous analyses (Cardon et al. 1994, 1995), selection for decreasing discriminant scores gave increasing evidence for linkage. This would support the idea that the gene is more common in more severely disabled readers.

While a p value of less than 0.05 is traditionally considered significant evidence against a null hypothesis, geneticists have generally agreed that a higher standard must be set for the acceptance of linkage, partially because of the great many tests often done as the entire genome is searched for linkage. Thomson, 1994, suggested three levels of significance and the requirements for replication: (1) weak linkage or association (<0.05) obtained in at least 3 independent data sets; or (2) moderate linkage (<0.01) obtained in at least 2 data sets; or (3) strong linkage (<0.001) in one, or in the overall, data set. Lander and

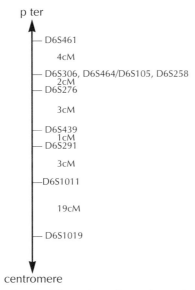

Figure 1.   Position of markers along chromosome 6p21.3. Genetic distances are given in centimorgans.

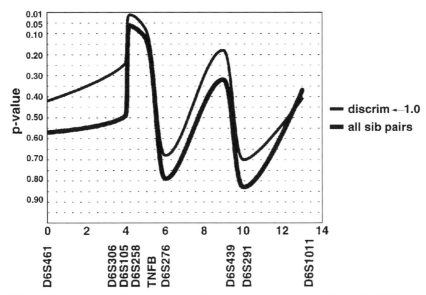

Figure 2.   *p* values for two-point linkage analysis of reading disability to markers on chromosome 6*p*21.3. One curve shows the analysis including all sib pairs in the study, and the second shows only those pairs in which at least one sib had a discriminant score of less than –1.0.

Kruglyak (1995) contended that, when a full genome search is done, the appropriate significance level for suggestive linkage would be $<7 \times 10^{-4}$, for significant linkage $<2 \times 10^{-5}$, and for highly significant linkage $<3 \times 10^{-7}$. Since Grigorenko et al. (1997) have found a p value less than 0.005 for several markers in the same region, the two studies combined would fulfill Thomson's criteria for acceptance of linkage to this region. Neither of these studies was a full genome search, and to date, a full genome search for reading disability has not been reported.

The linkage results in this expanded population are quite similar to those previously reported in that the most likely interval containing the gene is in the vicinity of D6S105/464. Examination of the results provided by Grigorenko et al. (1997) also shows that the area of highest significance contained D6S306 and D6S464, although D6S105, which was reported separately and at that time was thought to be some distance away from D6S464, was not significant. Since a different set of primers would have been used for the typing of D6S105 and D6S464, amplifying a slightly different section of DNA, the D6S105 marker may not have been as informative for linkage as D6S464 in their population of families, even though both markers appear to cover the same locus.

It should be noted that while a significant p value indicates that a marker is linked to RD, the relative p value for several significant markers is not a reliable indicator that the gene is closer to one marker than to another. That is, the fact that the p values for D6S258 are slightly higher than those for D6S105 does not mean that the gene is closer to D6S258, since significance levels are also influenced by how informative each marker is in that particular population. For example, if the parents and siblings in a family all have the same genotype, the identity by descent of the particular alleles cannot be determined, and that sibling pair cannot contribute to the overall significance level. In smaller samples and lower significance levels, such variation may have more of an effect on the relative magnitude of the p values. Larger samples are necessary to reliably define the region most likely to contain the gene.

The results of the Transmission Disequilibrium Test in the GAS package further support the linkage through association analysis. Significant association was found with one allele of the marker D6S306. Since this test uses only heterozygous parents (two different alleles at a marker), the sample size is small; for example, even though the significance level was 0.037 for D6S06, this represented only 5 observations in which a parent had a #6 allele at that marker. In all 5, the #6 allele was transmitted. While the results of these analyses were consistent with the linkage results to the other markers in this tight linkage group, increasing sample sizes may modify the results.

Overall, the results of the current study continue to support the existence of a gene influencing reading disability in a small region of chromosome 6p21.3. We are continuing to expand the study population and will examine the effects of additional reading disability phenotypes to see if a particular phenotype is especially influenced by that gene. We will also type additional markers to determine the boundaries of the critical region containing this gene. Once the location of the gene is refined to a small enough region (ideally, less than 1 centimorgan), additional molecular and genetic techniques exist to find the gene itself. This is more difficult for traits such as reading disability, where a gene may be present in an individual but not always cause the condition; and conversely, the condition may exist without the particular gene. Identification of "candidate genes," known to be in the region and to have a function that might be related to reading, will be critical. Fortunately, as more genes are identified through the Human Genome Project and related research, more candidate genes will be available for analysis. Ultimately, functionally important mutations in a particular candidate gene must be found significantly more often in several different populations of disabled readers in order to determine that the gene has an influence on reading.

REFERENCES:

Cardon, L. R. and Fulker, D. W. 1994. The power of interval mapping of quantitative trail loci, using selected sib pairs. *American Journal of Human Genetics* 55:825–33.

Cardon, L. R., Smith, S. D., Fulker, D. W., Kimberling, W. J., Pennington, B. F., and DeFries, J. C. 1994. Quantitative trait locus for reading disability on chromosome 6. *Science* 266: 276–79.

Cardon, L. R., Smith, S. D., Fulker, D. W., Kimberling, W. J., Pennington, B. F., and DeFries, J. C. 1995. Quantitative trait locus for reading disability: A correction (letter). *Science* 268: 5217.

DeFries, J. C., Fulker, D. W., and LaBuda, M. C. 1987. Reading disability in twins: Evidence for a genetic etiology. *Nature* 329:537–39.

DeFries, J. C., and Gillis, J. J. 1993. Genetics of reading disability. In *Nature, Nurture, and Psychology*, eds. R. Plomin and G. McClearn. Washington, D.C.: APA Press.

Gilger, J. W. 1992. Genetics in disorders of language. *Clinics in Communication Disorders* 2:35–47.

Gilger, J. W., Borecki, I. B., DeFries, J. C., and Pennington, B. F. 1994. Commingling and segregation analysis of reading performance in families of normal reading probands. *Behavior Genetics* 24:345–55.

Grigorenko, E. L., Wood, F. B., Meyer, M. S., Hart, L. A., Speed, W. C., Shuster, A., and Pauls, D. L. 1997. Susceptibility loci for distinct components of developmental dyslexia on chromosomes 6 and 15. *American Journal of Human Genetics* 60:27–39.

Haseman, J. K., and Elston, R. C. 1972. The investigation of linkage between a quantitative trait and a marker locus. *Behavior Genetics* 2:3–19.

Kidd, K. K. 1993. Associations of disease with genetic markers: Déjà vu all over again. *American Journal of Medical Genetics (Neuropsychiatric Genetics)* 48:71–73.

Lander, E., and Kruglyak, L. 1995. Genetic dissection of complex traits: Guidelines for interpreting and reporting linkage results. *Nature Genetics* 11: 241–47.

Pennington, B. F., Gilger, J. W., Pauls, D. L., Smith, S. A., Smith, S. D., and DeFries, J. C. 1991. Evidence for dominant transmission of developmental dyslexia. *The Journal of the American Medical Association* 266:1527–34.

Smith, S. D. 1992. Identification of genetic influences. *Journal of Communication Disorders* 2:73–85.

Smith, S. D., Gilger, J. W., and Pennington, B. F. 1995. Dyslexia and other language/learning disorders. In *Emery and Rimoin's Principles and Practice of Medical Genetics, 3rd Edition*, eds. D. L. Rimoin, J. M. Conner, and R. Pyeritz. New York: Churchill Livingstone.

Spielman, R. S., McGinnis, R. E., and Ewens, W. J. 1993. Transmission test for linkage disequilibrium: The insulin gene region and insulin-dependent diabetes mellitus. *American Journal of Human Genetics* 52:506–16.

Thomson, G. 1994. Identifying complex disease genes: Progress and paradigms. *Nature Genetics* 8:108–10.

Chapter • 5

Early Identification of Children At Risk for Reading Disabilities
Phonological Awareness and Some Other Promising Predictors

Hollis S. Scarborough

"The greater becomes the volume of our sphere of knowledge, the greater also becomes its surface of contact with the unknown."

Jules Sageret

Research over the past two decades on the crucial role of phonological awareness in learning to read has greatly expanded "the volume of our sphere of knowledge." There is clear evidence that some degree of insight into the phonological structure of spoken words greatly enables a child to begin to discover the "alphabetic principle" (that printed letters ordinarily stand for phonemic segments of words), and that most children who have difficulty learning to read lack this insight (e.g., Adams and Bruck 1995; Brady and Shankweiler 1991; Liberman et al. 1974). Once the alphabetic principle has begun to be grasped, greater depths of phonological awareness are attained in conjunction with increasing mastery in the decoding of print, reflecting an apparent reciprocal relationship between the two developing abilities (e.g., Ehri and Wilce 1980, 1986; Perfetti et al. 1987). Not surprisingly, therefore, persistent weaknesses in both decoding and phonological awareness are defining characteristics of reading disability in both childhood and adulthood. (See Fowler and Scarborough 1993 for a review.) We also know that training novice readers and low achievers to attend to and manipulate phonemic segments, and to understand their relationship to letters, can facilitate reading acquisition (e.g., Blachman 1991; Torgesen in press). One current approach in circumventing dyslexia is to identify kindergartners who are weak in phonological awareness and provide them with such training.

As we have gained volumes of knowledge about phonological awareness, however, I think that our research efforts have also revealed how much more there is to understand about the etiology of dyslexia and the prediction of reading achievement; that is, the "surface of contact with the unknown" has also been enlarged. Without disagreeing with the insights gained about the role of phonological awareness, I think there is something more to be learned by looking at other findings from the recent literature on the prediction of reading (dis)abilities. That body of work indicates that, aside from phonological awareness, several other equally strong indicators of a young child's risk for developing reading problems exist. This information is potentially useful for improving methods for the early identification and treatment of at-risk children, for raising new questions to be pursued in future research, and for arriving, ultimately, at a comprehensive theoretical explanation of reading disabilities.

PREDICTING FUTURE READING ACHIEVEMENT FROM KINDERGARTNERS' CHARACTERISTICS AND SKILLS

Once a child has received some formal instruction in school and has begun to learn to read, the best predictor of *future* reading attainment is how well the child can already read. As shown in table I, the temporal stability of reading achievement scores is considerable. Children who succeed early on rarely stumble later; and a majority of children who initially have difficulty tend to remain behind their classmates, even though many receive remedial help in reading. Before children are able to read, predicting future achievement is a more challenging problem. At about the time they enter kindergarten, wide differences among children, many of whom have minimal or nonexistent reading skills, exist. Prediction research indicates that some of these differences among kindergartners are more informative than others about future academic success. I will begin by considering several kinds of demographic and home background variables, and then focus on differences in children's abilities and knowledge in various domains.

Demographic and Home Background Differences

Sex. Historically, many more boys than girls have been identified by schools and clinics as having reading disabilities. This imbalance appears to arise mainly from ascertainment biases on the part of those who make referrals because on objective tests of reading ability, nearly as many girls as boys earn low scores (e.g., Naiden 1976; Shaywitz et al. 1990). Accordingly, a kindergartner's sex has generally been found to be a very weak predictor of future reading achievement in most longitudinal studies (e.g., Badian 1994; Horn and O'Donnell 1984; Mann and Ditunno 1990; Scanlon and Vellutino 1996; Share et al. 1984). In short, the risk for developing a reading disability is only slightly higher for boys than girls.

Age for grade. Because eligibility for school entry is usually based on a chronological age cutoff, there is typically a 12-month age range

Table I. Temporal stability of reading ability differences and of reading disability classifications in studies that have assessed reading with the same test on at least two occasions for the same sample of children. (RD = reading disabled, by research criteria; NRD = not reading disabled.)

Sample	From Grade	To Grade	Time Interval	r	% RD Who Remain RD	% NRD Who Remain NRD
Badian (1988) 98%	3rd	8th	5 years	—		74%
Butler (1988)	3rd	6th	3 years	.77		
	3rd	8th	5 years	.78		
Butler et al. (1985)	1st	2nd	1 year	.69		
	1st	3rd	2 years	.69		
	1st	6th	5 years	.64		
	2nd	3rd	1 year	.88		
	2nd	6th	4 years	.78		
	3rd	6th	3 years	.86		
Juel (1988)	1st	4th	3 years	—	88%	87%
McGee et al. (1988)	1st	7th	6 years	—		56%
Satz et al. (1981)	2nd	5th	3 years	—	87%	76%
Scarborough (1995)	2nd	8th	6 years	.72	58%	97%
Shaywitz et al. (1992)*	1st	3rd	2 years	.67	47%	97%
	3rd	5th	2 years	.63	47%	92%
Wright et al. (1991)	2nd	7th	5 years	—	67%	91%

*Discrepancy of reading from aptitude, rather than absolute reading level, was examined in this study.

within a given entering class. Concerned that maturational differences could place their children at a disadvantage, parents whose children are the youngest in the class sometimes choose to defer the start of schooling (a practice often termed "red shirting") in the hope that their children will have more successful academic (and social and athletic) careers if they are among the oldest in the class. It appears, however, that with regard to reading attainment, maturational differences tend to be fully sorted out by the end of second grade, by which time age-for-grade is essentially unrelated to achievement scores (e.g., Morrison, Griffith, and Alberts 1997). It is not surprising, therefore, that weak correlations between age-for-grade and achievement have generally been obtained in longitudinal prediction studies (e.g., Badian 1994; Busch 1980; Horn and O'Donnell 1984; Scanlon and Vellutino 1996; Weller, Schnittjer, and Tuter 1992). Younger chronological age relative to classmates does not appear to be an important risk factor.

Socioeconomic and sociocultural differences. Household income and parents' education and occupations are conventional indices of the socioeconomic status (SES) of a family. Low SES is commonly associated with a broad array of environmental circumstances that may be detrimental to the development of young children, from poor prenatal and pediatric health care to the quality of neighborhood schools. Each of these associated conditions, on its own, could potentially place a child at risk for reading difficulties. Teasing them apart is virtually impossible, and this should be borne in mind when considering the evidence of SES as a predictor of reading disabilities.

The relationship between SES and reading achievement is more complex than is generally realized. In particular, the degree of risk associated with the SES of an *individual* child's family is considerably lower than the degree of risk associated with the SES level of a *group* of students attending a particular school. White (1982) reviewed 93 studies in which two pieces of information—the average SES of each school, and the average achievement level of the students attending that school—were obtained for a large sample of schools. He calculated that the average size of the correlation between SES and achievement was .68, which is very substantial. In contrast, in 174 studies that measured achievement scores and SES individually for all children in a large sample, an average correlation of only .23 was obtained. Similarly low estimates have been reported in numerous other studies of SES as an individual risk factor (e.g., Alwin and Thornton 1984; Estrada et al. 1987; Horn and O'Donnell 1984; Richman, Stevenson, and Graham 1982; Rowe 1991; Share et al. 1984; Walberg and Tsai 1985). In other words, *within a* particular school or district, socioeconomic differences among children are only weakly predictive of differing levels of reading achievement.

Home literacy environment. The finding that there are much weaker correlations between SES and achievement when child-to-child variation is analyzed than when school-to-school differences are examined may suggest that the quality of schooling is largely responsible for the low achievement typically shown by students from low SES families and communities; if so, preventing the reading problems of these children would best be addressed by improving their schools. On the other hand, it has been hypothesized that there are real socioeconomic or sociocultural differences that contribute to achievement differences, but that these dimensions of differences are not adequately captured by demographic measures such as income and parental education. Instead, characteristics of the home environment that are directly related to the acquisition of literacy skills and attitudes may be better predictors of an individual child's risk for reading difficulties. Hess and Holloway (1984) emphasized several such family practices: parental reading habits; reading to children by adults; stimulating verbal interactions between adults and children; high parental expectations of achievement by their children; and availability of reading and writing materials.

When these and other aspects of the home literacy environment have been investigated in relation to reading achievement in studies of elementary school children, the estimated strength of the relationship has been quite inconsistent, and weaker in the early grades than in older samples (e.g., Iverson and Walberg 1982; Rowe 1991; Walberg and Tsai 1985; White 1982). Of greater relevance to the focus of this chapter—the early prediction of reading disability—are longitudinal studies that have measured various aspects of preschool or kindergarten children's home experiences (usually as reported by parents) and examined differences in relation to subsequent reading achievement scores in the primary school grades. In such studies, the amount of reading that parents do in the home has been a very weak predictor (e.g., DeBaryshe et al. 1991; Scarborough, Dobrich, and Hager 1991; Thomas 1984), but future reading achievement has been found to correlate reliably with the availability of reading materials in the home (median $r = .27$) and with library experiences (.17) (DeBaryshe 1993; Mason 1980; Mason and Dunning 1986; Share et al. 1984; Wells 1985). The amount and quality of parent-child book reading during the preschool years is the aspect of the home environment that has been studied most often; and two recent meta-analyses of the several dozen studies on this issue both concluded that the average magnitude of this correlation is about .28 or less (Bus, van IJzendoorn, and Pellegrini 1995; Scarborough and Dobrich 1994). Scarborough and Dobrich (1994) also observed that stronger correlations did not appear to be obtained when home literacy practices were looked at in combination, rather than singly, as predictors of reading. Therefore, while indicating that positive relationships exist between several aspects of the preschool home literacy environment and subsequent reading achievement, the findings are not strong enough to be of much practical use for identifying children who are at risk for reading disabilities.[1]

Familial incidence of dyslexia. Reading problems tend to run in families, and great strides have recently been made in teasing apart the genetic and environmental bases for this. (See Smith, this volume.) Several studies have attempted to estimate the degree of risk imposed on a child whose family includes one or two parents (and/or older siblings) with reading disabilities. The percentages of children from such families who turned out to have reading disabilities are listed in table II. Although there is considerable variation in the degree of estimated risk from study to study, this, in part, reflects differences in the criteria used to define reading disability in adults and children. All together, the results indicate that the incidence of reading disability in a child's immediate family clearly puts a child at increased risk for dyslexia. It is also clear, of course, that while many children from such families are likely to have difficulty learning to read, many will not. In order to predict individual outcomes, it is important to know what early characteristics of individual children are the most reliable and informative indicators of risk.

Individual Differences in Knowledge and Skill

As noted earlier, one approach to the prevention of reading problems that is gaining widespread attention is to identify kindergartners who are at greatest risk for unsuccessful reading acquisition and direct intervention efforts toward those children. Clearly, the success of such an approach will depend, in part, on the accuracy with which the risk status of young children can be determined. If the basis for identifying at-risk youngsters is overly inclusive (i.e., if the number of "false positive" prediction errors is high), the costs will be magnified by the

---

[1]In light of the generally weak correlations between home factors and later achievement found in most studies, it is difficult to interpret the more encouraging results of the one study in which the home environment was evaluated at much younger ages (12 and 24 months). Bradley and Caldwell (1984; Bradley, Caldwell, and Rock 1988) found that in their sample of 37 children, the HOME index was highly correlated with reading in first grade ($r = .56–65$) but not significantly in fourth grade ($r = .24$).

Table II. Estimates of Parent-to-Child Risk for Dyslexia

| Study | Diagnostic Criteria | | % of Children Affected |
	Parents	Children	
Badian (1988)	self-report	testing	23%
Finucci et al. (1985)	Gow School alumni	parent report	36%
Fowler and Cross (1986)	self-report	testing	33%
Gilger et al. (1991)			
Sample 1	self-report	testing	25–41%
Sample 2	self-report	testing	47–65%
Sample 3	self-report	testing	31–49%
Scarborough (1989)	self-report	school identif'n	42%
	self-report	testing	53%
	testing	school identif'n	43%
	testing	testing	62%

necessity of treating many more children than actually need any intervention. Furthermore, there may be unforseen consequences of labeling a large number of children "at risk" who would have acquired reading successfully without intervention. On the other hand, using an overly restrictive identification algorithm that yields large numbers of "false negative" errors will result in a failure to provide services to many children who need them. Minimizing both kinds of prediction errors, therefore, is an important concern in setting up procedures for identifying children who are at greatest risk for reading difficulties.

A great deal of information about the prediction of primary grade reading scores from earlier assessments has been amassed from longitudinal research during the past two decades.[2] The remainder of this chapter will be largely devoted to presenting a quantitative review of that body of work. In these studies, a sample of children has usually been assessed first during the kindergarten year (i.e., at about age 4.5 to 6 years, although some studies have begun testing during the year prior to kindergarten); and others (particularly from countries in which no reading instruction occurs before first grade) in the early months of the first grade. Most of this research has focused on "unselected" samples, although few of these have been truly population-representative. A few studies have included high-risk samples (e.g., clinic samples of children with early language impairment; children from low SES backgrounds; offspring of dyslexic parents), alone or in conjunction with

---

[2]Although many early prediction studies were carried out prior to the mid-1970s, the demands of today's primary curricula and the composition of the contemporary student body have changed enough since then that the relevance of the older studies may be reduced; this review is thus based primarily on more recent findings.

"control" groups; it is not yet clear whether particular factors are associated with the same degree of risk for all subgroups of children, although there is no evidence to the contrary. Many kinds of skills, attainments, and background differences have been investigated as prospective predictors of reading, and their correlations with future reading scores have usually been provided by the investigators (although, in a few studies, only classificatory or multivariate results have been reported). Therefore, for each predictor measure, I was able to estimate the average magnitude of its association with reading outcomes by aggregating findings across studies.

The criteria for inclusion in the analyses and the procedures for averaging correlation coefficients were as follows. All studies on the prediction of reading since 1976 that I could locate were included, providing that: (1) the sample size was 30 or larger; (2) at least one risk factor was assessed initially when the children were within ±1 year of beginning formal schooling in reading; and (3) at least one assessment of reading skill was made after one, two, or occasionally, three years of instruction. These criteria were met for 53 samples from 61 studies. If a word recognition outcome measure was obtained, its correlation with predictors was used; otherwise, a composite reading score or, rarely, a reading comprehension measure was accepted instead as the criterion variable. When more than one correlation value per risk factor was available in a given sample of children (because multiple reading assessments were conducted and/or because multiple measures of the predictor were used), the average correlation for the sample was used for aggregation. When correlations were averaged across studies, each research sample contributed only one, independent, observation.

The strengths of many kinds of predictor variables, alone and in combination, will be reviewed below. A summary comparison of the effects for different predictors is provided in table III. In addition, more detailed information about the aggregated data is provided in tables A-1 through A-7 of the Appendix .

Print-specific knowledge and skills. As already noted, reading ability itself is generally the best basis for predicting future reading scores of school children. Might this relationship extend downward to prediction from even earlier ages? Even before children can "read" (in the conventional sense), most have acquired some information about the purposes, mechanics, and component skills of the reading task. Especially now, opportunities for acquiring this information abound (e.g., daycare and preschool enrollment, exposure to educational television and software, engaging in joint book reading with parents), although not all children receive equal amounts of exposure to such sources. By the time children begin school, they vary considerably in how much they already know about books and reading.

Two main kinds of measures of developing literacy knowledge and skills have been used in prediction studies. The more traditional type includes "reading readiness" tests and the kindergarten and pre-kindergarten levels of standardized achievement batteries. These usually assess a variety of component skills thought to play a role in reading acquisition, such as: visual discrimination of letters or letter-like forms; discrimination of speech sounds; phonological sensitivity to the structure of spoken words (e.g., Which words begin with the same sound: *king, gate, corn?*); recognition or production of the names of letters; knowledge of the correspondences between letters and sounds (e.g., Which two spoken words would begin with the same first letter: *dog, doll, boat?*); and actual reading aloud of printed words. The other, more functional types of measures, such as Clay's (1979) test of print concepts, evaluates a child's knowledge about the purposes and mechanics of reading; for example, the child's understanding of why people read, how a book is manipulated, and the differences between print and pictures.

Table A-1 in the Appendix lists the correlations with future reading achievement obtained in predictive studies using these types of tests. For the more traditional "readiness" measures, the average correlation across the 22 recent samples in my analysis was .56, which is similar to the estimate of .50 that Hammill and McNutt (1981) arrived at for 19 samples from studies between 1950 and 1977. On the other hand, in the seven prediction studies to date that used the newer, more functional measures, results were somewhat mixed, with an average effect size of .46–.49. Higher correlations were obtained in the two samples in which both types of tests were given, suggesting that using this combined approach may be useful for attaining greater accuracy in identifying children at risk for reading disabilities, although this needs additional confirmation in future research.

Among the "readiness" skills that are traditionally evaluated, the one that appears to be the strongest predictor on its own is *letter identification*. The rightmost column of table A-1 shows the results for longitudinal studies since 1976 that have included this measure. Across these 24 research samples, the median correlation between letter naming scores and subsequent reading achievement is .53, with a mean of .52 (*SD* = .14). (Earlier prediction studies produced similar results; Jansky and de Hirsch 1972.) In other words, just measuring how many letters a kindergartner is able to name appears to be nearly as successful at predicting future reading as is giving a more comprehensive readiness battery.

Although not so strong as the temporal stability of reading scores from first grade onward (median r = .69; see table I.), the prediction of future reading by kindergarten measures of letter identification and other early reading skills is quite substantial, accounting for nearly a third of the variance in reading at grades one through three. Nevertheless, the predictive accuracy derived from using such readiness measures alone is lower than desirable for practical purposes. In Scanlon and Vellutino's (1996) very large, district-wide sample, letter knowledge at the start of kindergarten was correlated .59 with reading test scores, and .61 with teacher ratings of reading skill, at the end of first grade. However, when letter identification was used to classify kindergartners as "at risk" or not, many errors occurred in predicting which children would end up in the bottom 20% in first grade reading. Distribution of prediction errors was contingent upon how strict the risk classification criteria were. For example, when a rather strict criterion was adopted, i.e., when letter identification scores were used to identify only the bottom 10% of kindergartners as "at risk," then 83.2% of the first grade outcomes of the approximately 1000 children would have been correctly predicted on the basis of letter knowledge. Of the 100 kindergartners who would have been identified as most at risk (and who would have been presumably targeted to receive intervention), fully 37% would have turned out not to have reading difficulties. Furthermore, of the 900 children deemed not to be at risk on the basis of letter knowledge, fully 131 (14.5%) would have developed reading problems by the end of first grade. In other words, only about one third of the children who became the poorest readers would have been selected initially for early intervention. When a more lenient criterion was used to classify kindergartners (25% rather than 10% were considered "at risk"), then the "negative predictive power" (NPP—the proportion of not-at-risk designees who did not become poor readers) would rise from 85.5 to 90%; but the overall accuracy of prediction would decrease slightly to 79.5% making the "positive prediction power" (PPP—the percentage of children in the at-risk group who indeed became poor readers) drop substantially, with less than half of the "at risk" group actually expected to develop reading difficulties.

To increase the accuracy with which the risk status of kindergartners can be identified, it is probably necessary to assess other individual risk factors that may provide additional information about how readily a child is likely to learn to read. The relative predictive strengths will be reviewed for phonological awareness and 18 other kinds of abilities, many of which have been hypothesized to contribute to, and perhaps be necessary for, successful reading acquisition.

Phonological awareness.   Phonological awareness, or phonological sensitivity, is the ability to attend explicitly to the phonological structure of spoken words, rather than just to their meanings and syntactic roles. This is a particularly interesting skill to look at as a predictor of reading because, as mentioned earlier, training young children to attend to subsyllabic components, particularly phonemic segments, of words has been shown to facilitate their discovery of the regular correspondences between printed letters and phonemes they represent in alphabetic writing systems like English, suggesting that phonemic awareness plays a causal role in reading acquisition.

The predictive correlation of phonological awareness to subsequent reading has been examined in 27 research samples from 24 studies, whose results are listed in the first column of correlation coefficients in table A-2.[3] While a few studies have reported extremely high correlations, the more typical findings have clustered in the .37 to .46 range, so the mean effect (.46) exceeds the median (.42). On the average, phonological awareness accounts for less variance in future reading scores (18–21%) than does letter identification or traditional readiness scores (27–31%).

When classificatory analyses are conducted, phonological awareness in kindergarten appears to have the unfortunate tendency to be more of a successful predictor of future *superior* reading than of future reading *problems*. That is, among children who have recently begun, or will soon begin, kindergarten, few of those with strong phonological awareness skills will stumble in learning to read, but many of those with weak phonological sensitivity will go on to become adequate readers. Moreover, as was described earlier for letter identification, if classification criteria are adjusted to increase the positive prediction power and reduce "false positive" errors, overall prediction accuracy tends to drop, so that more children who will become poor readers fail to meet the risk criterion. The following three examples illustrate this tendency. First, an analysis of the data from Bradley and Bryant's (1983) landmark study was described in their subsequent book (Bradley and Bryant 1985, pp. 101–105). Depending on the reading test used (Neale or Schonell), the overall accuracy in predicting reading status from prior phonological awareness (each adjusted for age and IQ) was 80% to 82%. Of the 25 children who were initially weakest in phonological awareness, only 24% to 28% turned out to be poor readers; and of the remaining 291 children, 14% to 15% developed reading problems.

---

[3]Because phonological awareness tasks that tap only a syllabic level of segmentation (e.g., syllable counting/tapping measures) have generally been less well correlated with later reading, results for such measures were not included in this analysis (table A-2).

Similarly, in a follow-up study of 41 language-impaired kindergartners, Catts (1991) found that a phoneme deletion task correctly classified 76% of the children with regard to their reading status at the end of first grade. (Another phonological awareness measure, requiring blending, was a bit less successful, predicting only 71% of outcomes in the sample.) Of the 25 children designated as "at risk" on the basis of their poor phonological awareness, 17 (68%) became poor readers but 8 (32%) did not; of the 16 "not at risk" children, 13% turned out to have reading problems despite their strong prior phonological awareness skills. The picture was much the same in the small study that yielded the highest correlation (.75) between phonological awareness skills (Mann 1984). The 12 kindergartners who became "poor" readers and the 22 who became "average" readers did about equally poorly on the phonological awareness test ($M = 0$% and 5% correct, respectively), while the 10 youngsters who became good readers did considerably better (33% correct). In other words, it is this large difference in phonological awareness between the highest-achieving group and the other groups (rather than the tiny difference between the two lower-achieving groups) that primarily underlies the correlational results.

Despite the theoretical importance of phonological awareness for learning to read, measures of this skill among 4.5- to 6-year-olds do not appear to predict subsequent reading achievement particularly well. This is mainly because at about the time of the onset of schooling, so many children who will go on to become normally achieving readers have not yet attained much, if any, appreciation of the phonological structure of oral language, making them nearly indistinguishable, in this regard, from children who will indeed encounter reading difficulties down the road.

Speech perception and production. Because phonological awareness is crucial for reading acquisition, yet, on its own, is only a moderately successful predictor of the future reading problems of kindergartners, the question can be raised as to whether deficiencies in phonological awareness might grow out of more basic deficits in phonological skills that develop from birth through the preschool years (Fowler 1991). For instance, perhaps children who have a better mastery of phonology—as exhibited by their ability to articulate speech sounds clearly and to hear spoken words accurately—can more readily gain a metalinguistic appreciation of the phonological structure of words. Moreover, Tallal (e.g., Tallal and Stark 1982) has further hypothesized that more fundamental weaknesses in auditory temporal processing may underlie speech perception deficits, ultimately resulting in reading disabilities.

Perceptual deficits have been observed in some, but not all, children with reading disabilities (For reviews see McBride-Chang 1995; Studdert-Kennedy and Mody 1995; and Watson and Miller 1993).

Several longitudinal prediction studies have examined kindergartners' receptive and productive phonological abilities in relation to future reading achievement, summarized in the last two columns of table A-2. From the available data, neither speech perception (median r = .23) nor speech production (.25), measured at about the time children enter school, appears to be a particularly useful predictor of subsequent reading differences.

General ability (IQ). Historically, the purpose of IQ tests was to assess scholastic aptitude, particularly to identify children who were likely to have difficulties in academic achievement. While the interpretation and use of IQ tests have changed considerably over time, the fundamental relationship between general intellectual abilities, especially verbal abilities, and achievement would be expected to hold; indeed, the predictive validity of such tests rests largely on such correlations. During the elementary school years, concurrently measured IQ and reading scores are reliably correlated. In Hammill and McNutt's (1981) meta-analysis, for instance, median correlations averaged over about a dozen studies were .44 for Full-Scale IQ, .42 for Verbal IQ, and .31 for Performance (nonverbal) IQ scores from the WISC, and .46 with scores on the Stanford-Binet. Stanovich, Cunningham, and Cramer's (1984) analyses of a larger sampling of studies suggested, furthermore, that concurrent IQ-reading correlations tend to be somewhat weaker during the primary grades (.30–.50) than at older ages (.45–.65).

Several longitudinal prediction studies have measured IQ at about age 4.5 to 6 years, primarily with the WISC-R, the WPPSI, or the McCarthy Scales of Preschool Abilities. As shown in table A-3, reading achievement was moderately well predicted by both Full-Scale IQ (mean r = .41) and Verbal IQ (.37), but less well by Performance IQ (.26) in these studies.

Vocabulary and naming abilities. Many researchers have used *receptive vocabulary* measures, such as the Peabody Picture Vocabulary Test, as a surrogate for general verbal ability in prediction studies. On each trial of such tests, the child must indicate which of several pictures best corresponds to the word (usually a noun, adjective, or gerund) spoken by the examiner. A long series of items of increasing difficulty is available, and testing terminates when the child's vocabulary level is exceeded. Correlations between kindergarten receptive vocabulary scores and subsequent reading scores in 19 prediction studies are listed in the first column of coefficients in table A-4. The distribution is negatively skewed, so the mean effect size (.33) differs somewhat from the median (.38), which resembles that for Verbal IQ.

Fewer prediction studies have examined expressive vocabulary, often called *confrontation naming*. On such measures as the Boston Naming Test, the child is shown a series of drawings of objects, and is asked to name each one. Compared to receptive tests, these measures place greater demands on accurate retrieval of stored phonological representations of lexical items, and on the formulation and production of spoken responses. Stimuli for confrontation naming tasks are presented with increasing difficulty, so that later items are readily recognizable objects whose names are not used very frequently. Some examples illustrating the range of difficulty on the Boston Naming Test are: whistle, seahorse, harmonica, escalator, funnel, and palette. Concurrent correlations of confrontation naming skill with reading, but not with attentional or mathematical problems, have been observed in numerous school-aged samples (e.g, Denckla and Rudel 1976a; Felton et al. 1987; Wolf 1991; Wolf and Goodglass 1986). To my knowledge, however, only five kindergarten prediction studies have included confrontational naming measures in the predictor battery. The magnitude (mean $r = .45$) and consistency of the results of those studies (listed in the second column of table A-4) suggest that naming vocabulary may be a reliable predictor of future reading success that has too often been overlooked by researchers.

Not just the accuracy of name production but also its speed can be measured. In *rapid serial naming* tasks, large arrays of highly familiar stimuli are presented, and the child is asked to name all of the items as quickly as possible. For instance, on the most widely used task of this sort, Denckla and Rudel's (1976b) Rapid Automatized Naming test, each 5 x 10 array contains ten recurrences, in random order, of a set of five items (pictured objects, color patches, digits, and letters). Each array can typically be named in about one minute or less, even by young children. Rapid serial naming speed has been shown to correlate with concurrent and future reading ability, but not with IQ, in several dozen studies of school children (e.g., Ackerman, Dykman, and Gardner 1990; Bowers and Swanson 1991; Cornwall 1992; Denckla and Rudel 1976b; Felton et al. 1987; Spring and Davis 1988; Wolf and Obregon 1991). Somewhat weaker associations with reading are obtained when "discrete" naming (response time to name an individual stimulus) rather than "serial" naming is measured, suggesting that the naming speed problems of poor readers involve more than just difficulty in retrieving and producing item names. However, a full understanding of the relationship between speed naming and reading remains to be determined. Recent evidence suggests, furthermore, that rapid serial naming speed may be an especially good predictor of subsequent progress once a child has developed a reading problem in the primary grades (Korhonen 1991; Lovett 1995; Meyer et al. in press; Scarborough 1995).

As a kindergarten predictor, rapid serial naming is of particular interest in light of the recent "double deficit" hypothesis, advanced by Bowers and Wolf (1993) and Wolf (in press), that reading disability can stem from either of two core deficits—phonological awareness or naming speed—and that the most severe reading problems result from the occurrence of both weaknesses. Rapid serial naming measures have been included as predictors in 14 longitudinal studies of kindergarten samples. As shown in the last two columns of table A-4, the average correlations between kindergartners' naming speeds and their later reading scores were quite similar when the arrays to be named included alphanumeric symbols (digits or letters) or nonsymbolic stimuli (colors or objects). Overall, the median correlation of rapid serial naming speed with reading was .40 and the mean was .38 in the 14 studies to date.

Other aspects of language comprehension and production. Spoken language and reading have much in common. As long as the printed words can be efficiently recognized, comprehension of the connected text will depend heavily on the reader's oral language abilities, particularly on his or her understanding of syntactic and semantic relationships among the morphemes, words, and phrases. Indeed, many early research reports called attention to the differences between good and poor readers in their comprehension and production of structural relations within spoken sentences.

As shown in table A-5, numerous longitudinal prediction studies have included measures of semantic, morphological, and syntactic skills of kindergartners. (Rarely, however, have different researchers used the same measures of these abilities, unfortunately.) The highest average correlation (.46–.47) has been found when a broad composite index of language abilities has been used, but only four studies have taken this approach so the findings should be considered promising but not definitive. Receptive (sentence comprehension) measures that emphasized the understanding of complex syntactic and morphological forms have been more successful predictors (average $r \le .38$) than other (or unspecified) kinds of receptive measures (.24–.25), and about equally strong predictors of reading as expressive (production) measures (.32–.37), which include mean length of utterance, sentence completion, morphological cloze tasks, and others. It should be recalled that the goal in these studies has been to predict reading achievement during the first few school grades, when the emphasis is primarily upon the acquisition of word recognition and decoding skills rather than on the comprehension of challenging material. In view of that, it is perhaps somewhat surprising that these kindergarten language measures, especially the broad composite indices, yield such respectable correlations with early reading. Nevertheless, from the practical standpoint of identifying individual children at highest risk for reading difficulties, it would seem that several predictor variables reviewed earlier appear to be more useful.

Verbal Memory.   The ability to retain verbal information in working memory is essential for reading and learning, so it might be expected that verbal memory measures would be effective predictors of future reading achievement. As shown in the last two columns of table A-5, many prediction studies have included such measures within their predictor batteries. From the results of those studies, it is quite clear that on the average, kindergartners' abilities to repeat sentences (e.g., on the WPPSI Sentence Imitation subtest) or to recall a brief orally presented story are more strongly related to their future reading achievement ($r = .45$–$.49$) than are their scores on digit span, word span, and pseudo-word repetition measures ($r = .31$–$.33$). One might speculate that the former type of measure, which is among the best of the predictors reviewed so far, gains power by tapping both memory and sentence processing abilities.

Visual and motor skills.   Learning to read requires that the child be able to perceive and discriminate letters of the alphabet, and learning to write further requires that these letter forms be reproduced by the child. Traditional readiness batteries typically included not just letter discrimination and writing measures (which will not be reviewed here) but also some measures of more basic visual and/or motor abilities. In both research and practice, these skills have been examined less often during the last two decades than before that time, as theoretical accounts of reading difficulties have shifted from an emphasis on sensorimotor deficits to an emphasis on language (especially phonological) weaknesses. As can be seen in table A-6, in the relatively few recent prediction studies that have examined these sorts of predictor variables, reading achievement has not been well predicted by measures of visual form discrimination (mean $r = .22$), visual-motor integration ($.16$), visual memory ($.31$), and motor skills ($.25$).

Summary: Comparison of Individual Risk Factors.   Evidence has been reviewed regarding the strengths of the correlations of many specific abilities of kindergartners with their reading skills one to three years later. A summary of the aggregated data on these zero-order effects is provided in table III, with predictor variables listed in decreasing order of strengths of correlations with future reading achievement.

Not surprisingly, measures of skills that are directly related to reading and writing—including knowledge about letter identities, about letter-sound relationships, and about the mechanics and functions of book reading—have yielded the highest simple correlations with subsequent reading scores. Each of these predictors, on its own, has typically accounted for about 21% to 31% of the variance in later reading achievement. Among the other measures that have been studied, four stand out as the strongest predictors of reading, each accounting for about 18% to 24% of the variance in later achievement scores: confrontation naming (expressive vocabulary); general language ability; sentence/story recall; and phonological awareness. Somewhat weaker effects (10–17% of reading variance) have been obtained for an-

Table III. Correlations of Individual Risk Factors with Future Reading Achievement: Summary

Predictor	# of Samples	median *r*	mean *r*	*SD*
Print-Specific Knowledge/Skills:				
Early Reading ("Readiness")	21	.56	.57	.12
Letter Identification alone	24	.53	.52	.14
Concepts of Print	7	.49	.46	.20
Non-Print-Specific Abilities:				
Confrontation Naming	5	.49	.45	.07
Sentence/Story Recall	11	.49	.45	.12
General Language Index	4	.47	.46	.15
Phonological Awareness	27	.42	.46	.13
Full-Scale IQ	11	.38	.41	.14
Verbal IQ	12	.38	.37	.11
Receptive Vocabulary	20	.38	.33	.17
Rapid Serial Naming	14	.40	.38	.09
Receptive Language (Syntax)	9	.40	≤.37	n.a.
Expressive Language Production	11	.37	.32	.16
Verbal Memory (Words, Digits)	18	.33	.33	.17
Visual Memory (Forms)	8	.28	.31	.12
Motor Skills	5	.26	.25	.09
Performance IQ	8	.25	.26	.11
Receptive Language (Semantic)	11	25	.24	.17
Speech Production	4	.25	n.a.	n.a.
Speech Perception	11	.23	.22	.09
Visual Discrimination	5	.20	.22	.15
Visual-Motor Integration	6	.13	.16	.12

other six predictors, all measures of general ability and various narrower facets of language skill. Weaker average correlations have been obtained for the nine other kindergarten abilities that have been examined, including speech production and perception, visual and verbal short-term memory measures, and other nonverbal abilities.

As noted earlier, however, even the best of these measures is not sufficiently discriminative on its own to insure the accurate early identification of children at greatest risk for reading difficulties. Too many errors of prediction ("false positives" and/or "false negatives," depending on the cut-off criterion chosen) will occur when one attempts to classify at-risk children on the basis of measures that account for only about a third or less of the variance in future reading. One approach to improving the accuracy of prediction is to try to combine predictor variables so that their cumulative strength exceeds the degree of prediction afforded by any one of them on its own. Research along these lines is reviewed next.

Combining Individual Risk Factors to Improve Prediction

Many researchers have examined the combined effects of several or many predictors of reading, with the results of such multivariate analyses summarized in table A-7. The first ten studies listed in the table provide data from school- or population-representative samples; the last four, provided mainly for comparison purposes, are based on samples from two special populations: samples of children who had received preschool diagnoses of language impairment (discussed in more detail later), and samples in which children with a family history of reading problems were deliberately over-represented. It should be noted, further, that the most successful prediction study listed in the table (Hurford et al. 1994) differs from the others in that the initial assessments were conducted during the fall of first grade, rather than in early kindergarten. Because my main concern is with predicting outcomes from kindergarten data, the other nine studies will be the focus of the following discussion.

In six of those nine studies, the predictor battery included letter identification and/or other measures of early literacy knowledge and skills (letter-sound knowledge, word recognition, concepts of print, teacher ratings, writing). Five included at least one measure of phonological awareness; four included an IQ score; and three included a verbal memory measure. Other predictors (rapid serial naming, other oral language skills, numerical knowledge, visual/visual-motor abilities, demographic variables) were included in two or fewer of the analyses. In some studies, the researchers assessed many other skills that turned out not to make a significant contribution to the prediction of reading, and are, therefore, not listed in the table (e.g., perceptual skills, demographic variables, home literacy environment measures, and others). But some of the apparently strongest bivariate predictors, according to the preceding section of this chapter (i.e., sentence/story recall, confrontation naming, and broad language indices) were rarely assessed in these studies; so their potential contributions to prediction when combined with other variables remain unknown.

In seven of the nine studies, researchers conducted multiple regression analyses, yielding R and R^2 values as summary statistics of the strengths of the relationship between kindergarten measures and later reading achievement. R^2 ranged from .41 to .71, with an average of 57% of the variance in reading scores accounted for by the analysis (mean r = .75). In comparison, the mean effect size for readiness tests alone was considerably lower (mean r = .57, table A-1), indicating that adding other kinds of measures to the predictor set can effectively strengthen the prediction.

Classificatory analyses were conducted in six of the nine studies. As shown in the last five columns of table A-7, the percentage of children whose reading outcome status (reading disabled or nondisabled) was correctly predicted by kindergarten risk status (based on the predictor battery) ranged from 80% to 92%, with a mean of 89%. These prediction analyses tend to achieve high specificity (i.e., on the average, 91% of nondisabled readers had been classified as "not at risk" in kindergarten), but somewhat lower sensitivity (i.e., on the average, only 78% of dyslexic children had been classified initially as "at risk"). Negative predictive power ranged from 91% to 99%, with a mean of 96%; in other words, on the average, the proportion of "not at risk" children who, nevertheless, developed reading problems was only 4%. Positive predictive power, however, ranged from 31% to 75%, with a mean of only 55%; that is, the proportion of at-risk children, who turned out not to have reading difficulties, was substantial (45%) and was not markedly lower than when predictions were based on letter identification or phonemic awareness alone, as described earlier.

A Special Case: Preschoolers with Specific Early Language Impairments.

Both the bivariate and multivariate results of prediction studies are consistent with the view, held by most researchers for the past two decades, that weakness in some sort of verbal/language skill underlies reading disabilities. If so, preschoolers with clinically diagnosed "specific early language impairments" (SELI) might be especially

likely to develop reading disabilities. There are more than a dozen follow-up studies of the later academic achievements of SELI samples.
Although the sampling criteria, the initial skill levels of the children,
and the measures of outcome status have not always been well specified, and have rarely been comparable from study to study, several
general trends are evident. First, about 40% to 75% of preschoolers
with SELI develop reading difficulties later, often in conjunction with
broader academic achievement problems (Aram and Hall 1989; Bashir
and Scavuzzo 1992). Second, regardless of the child's general cognitive abilities or therapeutic history, the risk for reading problems is
greatest when the child's impairment is severe in any aspect of language, broad in scope, and/or persistent over the preschool years.
Nevertheless, some children with only mild to moderate language delays, and who appear to overcome their spoken language difficulties
by the end of the preschool period, remain at greater risk than other
youngsters for the development of a reading disability (e.g., Bishop
and Adams 1990; Scarborough and Dobrich 1990; Stark et al. 1984).

Two recent longitudinal prediction studies are particularly informative about the prediction of reading for children with SELI based on
their observed differences at about the time of school entry (Bishop and
Adams 1990; Catts 1991, 1993). As summarized in table A-7, in both
studies 50% of the variance in reading achievement within the SELI sample could be accounted for by a small set of predictors measured at
about age five. The accuracy of prediction within these SELI samples
was lower than in the other studies listed in the table, perhaps due to
range restrictions since non-SELI children were not included in the samples. It is clear that children with SELI are at greatly elevated risk for
having difficulties in learning to read, and are a population that should
be specifically targeted to receive early intervention. Speech-language
professionals, to whom these children are typically referred, are probably the most appropriate individuals to provide this intervention. What
needs to be considered, however, is the most effective type of treatment
that should be given to these children at ages three to five years. Because
the causal relationships between SELI and RD are obscure (e.g., Kamhi
and Catts 1989), and because apparent (often spontaneous) recovery to
normal levels of language proficiency is commonly observed in this
group (Scarborough and Dobrich 1990), it may not be sufficient simply
to emphasize the improvement of articulatory, syntactic, and pragmatic
language skills, as is typically done. Although there is no available research or clinical evidence on this point, the correlational data for unselected populations suggest that the focus of early intervention might
fruitfully be expanded to include training in phonological awareness,
naming vocabulary, verbal memory, and print-specific skills.

Prediction of Reading From Differences Measured at Younger Ages

Compared to their classmates, some children's literacy-related skills are so weak when they enter school that one could say that the problem we are seeking to prevent *has already begun* by kindergarten. That is, those children are already behind in "reading achievement." It is, therefore, not surprising that some of the best predictors of future reading are skills that are closely tied to (or, arguably, actually products of) the process of learning to decode print; namely, letter identification, letter-sound knowledge, and phonological awareness. Moreover, sentence/story recall, vocabulary, and general language skills may also be enhanced, less directly, through reading and learning to read. If so, it might be desirable to try to prevent or reduce these differences among entering kindergartners by identifying children who are at risk of being at the bottom of the distribution when they begin kindergarten, and to intervene prior to school entry.

Although dozens of investigations on reading predictions from measures taken at about the time of school entry (4.5 to 6 years old) have been conducted, only a handful of longitudinal prediction studies have assessed children at younger ages (birth to age 4). Consistent with the theoretical consensus that some kinds of language deficits underlie most difficulties in learning to read, the main focus of all these investigations has been the development of linguistic and metalinguistic abilities in very young children, who are then followed through their early school years.

To my knowledge, only one study has directly examined reading prediction from developmental differences among infants. Shapiro et al. (1990) obtained reading scores at age 7.5 years for 227 children for whom pediatric records from birth to two years were available for numerous language and motor milestones, i.e., first word, 50-word vocabulary, 2-word utterances, sits unsupported, crawls, and walks. A composite measure of infant achievement was found to predict reading status (RD or not) with .73 sensitivity and .74 specificity. Individually, the "expressive" language milestones made a particularly strong contribution to prediction. Bayley infant IQ scores were about as good at predicting outcomes as the expressive language measure, but including IQ in the composite did not improve accuracy. Although not sufficiently accurate for practical use, this degree of predictive success is, nevertheless, remarkable in comparison to the results of the kindergarten studies described in table A-7.

Three studies have examined language and IQ as predictors in 2.5- to 4.5-year-old children. First, Walker et al. (1994) cumulatively monitored two aspects of emerging language (mean utterance length and number of vocabulary words produced) in monthly visits for a sample of 40 children aged 7 to 36 months, chosen as nationally representative demographically. Stanford-Binet IQ scores were also obtained at age three. They were able to follow 32 of the children during their early school years. The two early language measures, which were highly intercorrelated ($r = .85$), each correlated moderately well with reading scores in grades one through three ($r = .32$ to .63, mean = .46), as did the preschool IQ scores ($r = .33$ to .47, mean = .42).

Second, Bryant and his colleagues (Bryant, Maclean, and Bradley 1990; Bryant et al. 1990; Maclean, Bryant, and Bradley 1987) obtained scores for 64 children aged 40 to 41 months on a test of receptive vocabulary (EPVS), on the Expressive and Receptive portions of the Reynell language scale, on a measure of nursery rhyme recitation skill, and on a phonological awareness test (rhyme matching). Other phonological awareness measures were given at 44, 48, and 55 months, and a WPPSI IQ score was obtained at 51 months. Performance on reading tests, which were given at 75 and 79 months of age, was predicted by receptive vocabulary ($r = .43$), expressive language ability (.57), receptive language ability (.43), nursery rhyme recitation (.59), and IQ (.67). Correlations of the rhyme matching measure with later reading were not reported, and this measure was only weakly related (mean $r = .28$) to the tests of phonological awareness at 40 to 55 months, the last of which were strongly predictive of reading (mean $r = .66$), as was reported in table A-2.

Third, I (Scarborough 1991a, 1991b) obtained several language and IQ scores for a sample of 62 children between the ages of three and four years, about half of whom had parents and/or older siblings with reading problems, and examined their reading outcomes at the end of second grade. McCarthy IQ scores from ages 36 and 48 months correlated .33 and .36, respectively, with later reading. Scores on the receptive portion of the Northwestern Syntax Screening Test, also given at 36 and 48 months, were associated with reading to about the same degree ($r = .32$ and .34, respectively). Expressive vocabulary skill (Boston Naming Test) at age 42 months predicted reading more strongly ($r = .52$) than did receptive vocabulary (PPVT) scores at the same age ($r = .42$). In addition, for a subset of 52 children (20 from affected families who became disabled readers, 20 demographically similar nondisabled readers from unaffected families, and 12 who became good readers despite a family history of RD), measures of expressive phonological (pronunciation accuracy), syntactic (length/complexity of sentences), and lexical (word diversity) abilities were derived from naturalistic observations of children's language during play sessions at age 2.5 years (Scarborough 1990). The children who became poor readers were much weaker than the other groups on the syntactic and phonological measures at that early age.

What is most striking about the results of the preceding studies is that the magnitude of the bivariate correlations between reading and early preschool measures—taken three to five years prior to outcome assessments—is not markedly lower than that of the correlations of reading with kindergarten predictor scores for the same sorts of skills. Nevertheless, even if it might be possible to predict reading outcomes as successfully from age three as from age five, as these studies suggest, the practical utility of doing so is small. That is, in general it is probably not feasible to conduct population-wide screening of preschoolers for the purpose of identifying those who are at greatest risk for reading difficulties. Preschoolers with SELI and preschoolers with a family history of reading disability, however, are groups within the population for whom early detection and intervention are more realistic possibilities. If the future reading status of these children can be predicted from early measures of language and literacy skills, then it would be affordable potentially to assess that small subset of the population a year or two before kindergarten, and provide intervention to those with the weakest skills.

IMPLICATIONS FOR THEORY, RESEARCH, AND PRACTICE

Most contemporary accounts of the etiology of reading disabilities focus on phonological awareness as the predominant basis for the dyslexic child's difficulty in learning to read. As stated at the outset, on grounds of both logical importance (for grasping the alphabetic principle) and empirical evidence (from training studies), phonological awareness is the only predictor for which a strong claim for causality can be made. As has been reviewed, however, several other verbal abilities appear to be as strong or stronger than phonological awareness as predictors of the future reading achievement of kindergartners. Because correlation can never be presumed to imply causality, the etiological roles of these other predictor variables are open to question. The correlations can be interpreted differently based on different views about the underpinnings of dyslexia.

Within the prevailing "phonological" view, it is usually hypothesized that a deficit of some sort in more basic phonological processing is the root cause of dyslexia that impedes the attainment of phonological awareness, the proximal cause of reading failure. This more basic phonological deficit is hypothesized to have other ramifications too, some of which may also contribute to difficulties in learning to read, but many of which are largely irrelevant to the development of dyslexia despite their correlation with reading achievement. For example, verbal working memory weaknesses may arise if spoken material is poorly phonologically encoded for storage, and vocabulary acquisition may be impeded if the stored phonological representations of words are inaccurate or ill specified due to deficient encoding of speech. This provides a reasonable way of accounting for the results of prediction studies. That is, sentence/story recall may predict well because the phonological deficit weakens verbal working memory capacity; confrontation naming may predict well because lexical representations of names are degraded; and broad language indices may predict well because phonological difficulties interfere with the development of other aspects of language skill.

While plausible and admirably parsimonious, this account of the data is not yet airtight. For example, because they stem from a common core deficit, all of these successful predictors of reading should also correlate, at least moderately, with each other. This cannot be evaluated from the available data because few studies have included more than one of these measures and/or have reported the intercorrelations among predictor variables. Second, it is puzzling that other verbal working memory measures (digit span and word span) are not such strong predictors as sentence/story recall, even though the former would seem to require an even greater reliance on accurately encoded and retained phonological representations of the stimuli (due to the absence of contextual support). Similarly, it remains to be demonstrated convincingly that expressive vocabulary limitations have a phonological basis. In addition, the weak correlations of speech perception and speech production abilities with reading are also potentially inconsistent with the model, since these abilities would be expected to be compromised if a basic phonological deficit were present.

There are at least two other ways to account for the multiplicity of strong predictors. First, Wolf and Bowers (Bowers and Wolf 1993; Wolf in press) have put forth a "double deficit" hypothesis according to which either or both of two deficits (phonological awareness and naming speed) can underlie reading disability. While this particular combination does not receive strong support from the data reviewed above, some other sort of two-pronged causal model might work. Second, rather than hypothesizing there to be multiple causes of reading disabilities, one might postulate that there is a single core deficit, but one that is somewhat broader in scope than envisioned within the phonological core viewpoint (e.g., perhaps a language production deficit of some sort). Rather than postulating that sentence/story recall, confrontation naming, and broad language deficits all result from poor phonological encoding, one might see them as various manifestations of the core deficit that are evident somewhat earlier in life than is weak phonological awareness (Scarborough 1990, 1991a), and are thus good markers of risk but *not* necessarily proximal causes of difficulty in learning to read. In this sense, the etiology of dyslexia might be better envisioned as similar to that of the disease syphilis (in which a single underlying cause leads to a succession of potentially unrelated symptoms at different times) than to that of glaucoma (a simple causal chain).

Although it is interesting to entertain alternative hypotheses, the fact remains that the preponderance of the available data is reasonably consistent with the phonological core model. Nevertheless, I would like to encourage researchers to explore more deeply the etiological roles of the several promising non-phonological predictor variables identified in this review, with an eye toward testing between two or more theoretical viewpoints. In particular, tracing the developmental relationships among these skills, through the early preschool years as well as from kindergarten on, may be an especially fruitful approach.

With regard to the practical challenge of identifying kindergartners who are most at risk for developing reading problems, it is clear that a multivariate approach will produce greater accuracy than will reliance on any single test or measure. Even when multiple predictors are used to identify children at risk (table A-7), both sensitivity (78% on average) and positive predictive power (55%) have generally been lower than desirable for practical applications. That is, 22% of children who developed reading disabilities were not initially classified as at risk, and 45% of kindergartners meeting the risk criterion did not become disabled readers. This pattern of classification errors was quite similar across studies and suggests that some fair number of children who will develop reading disabilities do not obtain low enough scores in kindergarten to merit an "at risk" designation on the basis of the kinds of measures that have been used (most typically literacy-specific knowledge, phonological awareness, and IQ). Whether the inclusion of sentence/story recall, naming vocabulary, and broader language measures in kindergarten testing would help to pick up these cases is unknown, but it merits investigation on the basis of the strong bivariate results that have been obtained for those measures. Another possibility is that reading difficulties can stem from more than one underlying weakness, as suggested by the "double deficit" hypothesis. If so, disjunctive classification criteria (e.g., that which considers a child to be at risk if a low score is obtained on measure A or measure B or measure C, regardless of the overall level of performance by the child), rather than conjunctive criteria (as employed in current approaches), may be a means of obtaining higher prediction accuracy. It bears mentioning, however, that the average multiple correlation in the studies in table A-7 ($r = .75$) was about as strong as the year-to-year correlations obtained among reading achievement scores (table I) during the elementary school grades. It may be unreasonable, therefore, to expect to see more than modest increases in the strength of multivariate correlations, even if an optimal predictor battery is used and optimal risk classification rules are adopted.

Preparation of this chapter was supported, in part, by grant 12–FY95–0027 from the March of Dimes Birth Defects Foundation to the Research Foundation of the City University of New York and by program project grant HD01994 from NIH to Haskins Laboratories. Address for correspondence: Psychology Department, Brooklyn College of CUNY, Brooklyn NY 11210–2889. I also thank Joseph Torgesen and Carsten Elbro for providing unpublished details of their research findings.

REFERENCES

Adams, M., and Bruck, M. 1995. Resolving the "great debate." *American Educator* 19:7–20.

Ackerman, P. T., Dykman, R. A., and Gardner, M. 1990. Counting rate, naming rate, phonological sensitivity, and memory span: Major factors in dyslexia. *Journal of Learning Disabilities* 23:325–27.

Alwin, D. F., and Thornton, A. 1984. Family origins and the schooling process: Early versus late influence of parental characteristics. *American Sociological Review* 49:784–802.

Aram, D. M., and Hall, N. E. 1989. Longitudinal follow-up of children with preschool communication disorders: Treatment implications. *School Psychology Review* 18:487–501.

Badian, N. A. 1982. The prediction of good and poor reading before kindergarten entry: A 4-year follow-up. *Journal of Special Education* 16:309–18.

Badian, N. A. 1988. The prediction of good and poor reading before kindergarten entry: A nine-year follow-up. *Journal of Learning Disabilities* 21:98–123.

Badian, N. A. 1994. Preschool prediction: Orthographic and phonological skills, and reading. *Annals of Dyslexia* 44:3–25.

Badian, N. A. 1995. Predicting reading ability over the long term: The changing roles of letter naming, phonological awareness, and orthographic processing. *Annals of Dyslexia* 45:79–96

Bashir, A. S., and Scavuzzo, A. 1992. Children with language disorders: Natural history and academic success. *Journal of Learning Disabilities* 25:53–65.

Bishop, D. V. M., and Adams, C. 1990. A prospective study of the relationship between specific language impairment, phonological disorders and reading retardation. *Journal of Child Psychology and Psychiatry* 31:1027–50.

Blachman, B. A. 1991. Phonological awareness: Implications for prereading and early reading instruction. In *Phonological Processes in Literacy: A Tribute to Isabelle Y. Liberman*, eds. S. A. Brady and D. P. Shankweiler. Hillsdale, NJ: Lawrence Erlbaum Associates.

Blatchford, P., Burke, J., Farquhar, C., Plewis, I., and Tizard, B. 1987. Associations between pre-school reading related skills and later reading achievement. *British Educational Research Journal* 13(1):15–23.

Bowers, P. G., and Swanson, L. B. 1991. Naming speed deficits in reading disability. *Journal of Experimental Child Psychology* 51:195–219.

Bowers, P. G., and Wolf, M. 1993, March. A double-deficit hypothesis for developmental reading disorders. Presented to the Society for Research in Child Development, New Orleans.

Bowey, J. 1995. Socioeconomic status differences in preschool phonological sensitivity and first-grade reading achievement. *Journal of Educational Psychology* 87:476–87.

Bradley, L., and Bryant, P. E. 1983. Categorizing sounds and learning to read—a causal connection. *Nature* 301:419–21.

Bradley, L., and Bryant, P. E. 1985. Rhyme and reason in reading and spelling. *International Academy for Research in Learning Disabilities Monograph Series, No. 1.* Ann Arbor, MI: University of Michigan Press.

Bradley, R. H., and Caldwell, B. M. 1984. The relation of infants' home environments to achievement test performance in first grade: A follow-up study. *Child Development* 55:803–9.

Bradley, R. H., Caldwell, B. M., and Rock, S. L. 1988. Home environment and school performance: A ten-year follow-up and examination of three models of environmental action. *Child Development* 59:852–67.

Brady, S. A., and Shankweiler, D. P. (eds.) 1991. *Phonological Processes in Literacy.* Hillsdale, NJ: Lawrence Erlbaum Associates.

Bryant, P. E., Maclean, M., and Bradley, L. L. 1990. Rhyme, language, and children's reading. *Applied Psycholinguistics* 11:237–52.

Bryant, P. E., Maclean, M., Bradley, L. L., and Crossland, J. 1990. Rhyme and alliteration, phoneme detection, and learning to read. *Developmental Psychology* 26(3):429–38.

Bus, A. G., van IJzendoorn, M. H., and Pellegrini, A. D. 1995. Joint book reading makes for success in learning to read: A meta-analysis on intergenerational transmission of literacy. *Review of Educational Research* 65:1–21.

Busch, R. F. 1980. Predicting first grade reading achievement. *Learning Disabilities Quarterly* 3:38–48.

Butler, K. G. 1988. Preschool language processing performance and later reading achievement. In *Preschool Prevention of Reading Failure*, eds. R. L. Masland and M. W. Masland. Parkton, MD: York Press.

Butler, S. R., Marsh, H. W., Sheppard, M. J., and Sheppard, J. L. 1985. Seven-year longitudinal study of the early prediction of reading achievement. *Journal of Educational Psychology* 77:349–61.

Catts, H. W. 1991. Early identification of dyslexia: Evidence from a follow-up study of speech-language impaired children. *Annals of Dyslexia* 41:163–77.

Catts, H. W. 1993. The relationship between speech-language impairments and reading disabilities. *Journal of Speech and Hearing Research* 36:948–58.

Chew, A. L., and Lang, W. S. 1990. Predicting academic achievement in kindergarten and first grade from prekindergarten scores on the Lollipop test and Dial. *Educational and Psychological Measurement* 50:431–37.

Clay, M. 1979. *The Early Detection of Reading Difficulties: A Diagnostic Survey with Recovery Procedures.* Portsmouth, NH: Heinemann.

Colarusso, R., Gill, S., Plankenhorn, A., and Brooks, R. 1980. Predicting first-grade achievement through formal testing of 5-year-old high-risk children. *Journal of Special Education* 14:355–63.

Cornwall, A. 1992. The relationship of phonological awareness, rapid naming, and verbal memory to severe reading and spelling disabilities. *Journal of Learning Disabilities* 25:532–38.

Day, K. C., and Day, H. D. 1983. Ability to imitate language in kindergarten predicts later school achievement. *Perceptual and Motor Skills* 57:883–90.

DeBaryshe, B. D. 1993. Joint picture-book reading correlates of early oral language skill. *Journal of Child Language* 20:455–61.

DeBaryshe, B. D., Caulfield, M. B., Witty, J. P., Sidden, J., Holt, H. E., and Reich, C. E. 1991, April. The ecology of young children's home reading environments. Presented to the Society for Research in Child Development, Seattle.

Denckla, M. B., and Rudel, R. G. 1976a. Naming of object drawings by dyslexic and other learning disabled children. *Brain and Language* 3:1–15.

Denckla, M. B., and Rudel, R. G. 1976b. Rapid "automatized" naming (R.A.N.): Dyslexia differentiated from other learning disabilities. *Neuropsychologia* 14:471–79.

Ehri, L., and Wilce, L. S. 1980. The influence of orthography on readers' conceptualization of the phonemic structure of words. *Applied Psycholinguistics* 1:371–84.

Ehri, L., and Wilce, L. S. 1986. The influence of spellings on speech: Are alveolar flaps /d/ or /t/? In *Metalinguistic Awareness and Beginning Literacy*, eds. D. Yaden and S. Templeton. Exeter, NH: Heinemann.

Elbro, C., Borstrom, I., and Petersen, D. K. 1996, submitted. Predicting dyslexia from kindergarten: The importance of distinctness of phonological representations of lexical items.

Estrada, P., Arsenio, W. F., Hess, R. D., and Holloway, S. D. 1987. Affective quality of the mother-child relationship: Longitudinal consequences for children's school-relevant cognitive functioning. *Developmental Psychology* 23:210–15.

Felton, R. H. 1992. Early identification of children at risk for reading disabilities. *Topics in Early Childhood Special Education* 12:212–29.

Felton, R. H., Wood, F. B., Brown, I. S., and Campbell, S. K. 1987. Separate verbal memory and naming deficits in attention deficit disorder and reading disability. *Brain and Language* 31:171–84.

Feshbach, S., Adelman, H., and Fuller, W. 1977. Prediction of reading and related academic problems. *Journal of Educational Psychology* 69:299–308.

Finucci, J. M., Gottfredson, L., and Childs, B. 1985. A follow-up study of dyslexic boys. *Annals of Dyslexia* 35:117–36.

Flynn, T. M., and Flynn, L. A. 1978. Evaluation of the predictive ability of five screening measures administered during kindergarten. *Journal of Experimental Education* 46:65–70.

Fowler, A. E. 1991. How early phonological development might set the stage for phonemic awareness. In *Phonological Processes in Literacy*, eds. S. A. Brady and D. P. Shankweiler. Hillsdale, NJ: Lawrence Erlbaum Associates.

Fowler, A. E., and Scarborough, H. S. 1993. Should reading disabled adults be distinguished from other adults seeking literacy instruction? A review of theory and research. *Technical Report No. 93–7*, National Center for Adult Literacy, University of Pennsylvania.

Fowler, M. G., and Cross, A. W. 1986. Preschool risk factors as predictors of early school performance. *Developmental and Behavioral Pediatrics* 7:237–41.

Gilger, J. W., Pennington, B. F., and DeFries, J. C. 1991. Risk for reading disability as a function of family history in three family studies. *Reading and Writing: An Interdisciplinary Journal* 3:205–17.

Glazzard, M. 1977. The effectiveness of three kindergarten predictors for first grade achievement. *Journal of Learning Disabilities* 10:95–99.

Grogan, S. C. 1995. Which cognitive abilities at age four are the best predictions of reading ability at age seven? *Journal of Research in Reading* 18:24–31.

Gullo, D. G., Clements, D. H., and Robertson, L. 1984. Prediction of academic achievement with the McCarthy Screening Test and Metropolitan Readiness Test. *Psychology in the Schools* 21:264–69.

Hammill, D. D., and McNutt, G. 1981. *Correlates of Reading: The Consensus of Thirty Years of Correlational Research.* Austin, TX: PRO-ED.

Helfgott, J. 1976. Phonemic segmentation and blending skills of kindergarten children: Implications for beginning reading acquisition. *Contemporary Educational Psychology* 1:157–69.

Hess, R. D., and Holloway, S. 1984. Family and school as educational institutions. In *Review of Child Development Research*, ed. R. D. Parke. Chicago: University of Chicago Press.

Horn, W. F., and O'Donnell, J. P. 1984. Early identification of learning disabilities: A comparison of two methods. *Journal of Educational Psychology* 76:1106–18.

Hurford, D. P., Darrow, L. J., Edwards, T. L., Howerton, C. J., Mote, C. R., Schauf, J. D., and Coffey, P. 1993. An examination of phonemic processing abilities in children during their first-grade year. *Journal of Learning Disabilities* 26:167–77.

Hurford, D. P., Schauf, J. D., Bunce, L., Blaich, R., and Moore, K. 1994. Early identification of children at risk for reading disabilities. *Journal of Learning Disabilities* 27(6):371–82.

Iverson, B. K., and Walberg, H. J. 1982. Home environment and school learning: A quantitative synthesis. *Journal of Experimental Education* 50:144–51.

Jansky, J., and de Hirsch, K. 1972. *Preventing Reading Failure.* New York: Harper and Row.

Juel, C. 1988. Learning to read and write: A longitudinal study of 54 children from first through fourth grades. *Journal of Education Psychology* 80:437–47.

Juel, C., Griffith, P. L., and Gough, P. B. 1986. Acquisition of literacy: A longitudinal study of children in first and second grade. *Journal of Educational Psychology* 78(4):243–55.

Kamhi, A. G., and Catts, H. W. 1989. *Reading Disabilities: A Developmental Language Perspective.* Boston: College Hill.

Klein, A. E. 1980. Test-retest reliability and predictive validity of the Northwestern Syntax Screening Test. *Educational and Psychological Measurement* 40:1167–72.

Korhonen, T. T. 1991. Neuropsychological stability and prognosis of subgroups of children with learning disabilities. *Journal of Learning Disabilities* 24:48–57.

Levy, B. A., and Stewart, L. 1991, April. Early diagnosis and treatment of reading problems. Presented to the Society for Research in Child Development, Seattle.

Liberman, I. Y., Shankweiler, D., Fischer, F. W., and Carter, B. 1974. Explicit syllable and phoneme segmentation in the young child. *Journal of Experimental Child Psychology* 18:201–12.

Lindquist, G. T. 1982. Preschool screening as a means of predicting later reading achievement. *Journal of Learning Disabilities* 15:331–32.

Lovett, M. W. 1995, April. Remediating word identification deficits: Are the core deficits of developmental dyslexia amenable to treatment? Presented to the Society for Research in Child Development, Indianapolis.

Lundberg, I., Olofsson, A., and Wall, S. 1980. Reading and spelling skills in the first school years predicted from phonemic awareness skills in kindergarten. *Scandinavian Journal of Psychology* 21:159–73.

Lunzer, E. A., Dolan, R., and Wilkinson, J. E. 1976. The effectiveness of measures of operativity, language and short-term memory in the prediction of reading and mathematical understanding. *British Journal of Educational Psychology* 46:295–305.

Maclean, M., Bryant, P. and Bradley, L. 1987. Rhymes, nursery rhymes, and reading in early childhood. *Merrill-Palmer Quarterly* 33(3):255–81.

Mann, V. A. 1984. Longitudinal prediction and prevention of early reading difficulty. *Annals of Dyslexia* 34:117–36.

Mann, V. A., and Ditunno, P. 1990. Phonological deficiencies: Effective predictors of future reading problems. In *Perspectives on Dyslexia Vol. 2*, ed. G. Pavlidis. New York: John Wiley and Sons.

Mason, J. M. 1980. When do children begin to read: An exploration of four year old children's letter and word reading competencies. *Reading Research Quarterly* 15:203–27.

Mason, J. M. 1992. Reading stories to preliterate children: A proposed connection to reading. In *Reading Acquisition*, eds. P. B. Gough, L. C. Ehri, and R. Treiman. Hillsdale, NJ: Lawrence Erlbaum Associates.

Mason, J. M., and Dunning, D. 1986, April. Toward a model relating home literacy with beginning reading. Presented to the American Educational Research Association, San Francisco.

Massoth, N. A., and Levenson, R. L. 1982. The McCarthy Scales of Children's Abilities as a predictor of reading readiness and reading achievement. *Psychology in the Schools* 19:293–96.

McBride-Chang, C. 1995. Phonological processing, speech perception, and reading disabilties: An integrative review. *Educational Psychologist* 30: 109–21.

McCormick, C. E., Stoner, S. B., and Duncan, S. 1994. Kindergarten predictors of first grade reading achievement: A regular classroom sample. *Psychological Reports* 74:403–07.

McGee, R., Williams, S., and Silva, P. A. 1988. Slow starters and long-term backward readers: A replication and extension. *British Journal of Educational Psychology* 58:330–37.

Meyer, M. M., Wood, F. B., Hart, L. A., and Felton, R. H. in press. Selective predictive value of rapid automatized naming within poor readers. *Journal of Learning Disabilities*.

Morrison, F. J., Griffith, E. M., and Alberts, D. M. 1997. Nature-nurture in the classroom: Entrance age, school readiness, and learning in children. *Developmental Psychology* 33:254–62.

Muehl, S., and Di Nello, M. C. 1976. Early first-grade skills related to subsequent reading performance: A seven year follow-up study. *Journal of Reading Behavior* 8:67–81.

Naiden, N. 1976, February. Ratio of boys to girls among disabled readers. *Reading Teacher* 439–42.

Perfetti, C. A. , Beck, L., Bell, L., and Hughes, C. 1987. Phonemic knowledge and learning to read are reciprocal: A longitudinal study of first grade children. *Merrill-Palmer Quarterly* 33:283–319.

Randel, M. A., Fry, M. A., and Ralls, E. M. 1977. Two readiness measures as predictors of first- and third-grade reading achievement. *Psychology in the Schools* 14(1):37–40.

Richman, N., Stevenson, J., and Graham, P. J. 1982. *Preschool to School: A behavioral study*. London: Academic Press.

Rowe, K. J. 1991. The influence of reading activity at home on students' attitudes towards reading, classroom attentiveness and reading achievement: An application of structural equation modelling. *British Journal of Education Psychology* 61:19–35.

Rubin, R. A., Balow, B., Dorle, J., and Rosen, M. 1978. Preschool prediction of low achievement in basic skills. *Journal of Learning Disabilities* 11:62–65.

Satz, P., Fletcher, J., Clark, W., and Morris, R. 1981. Lag, deficit, rate, and delay constructs in specific learning disabilities: A reexamination. In *Sex Differences in Dyslexia*, eds. A. Ansara, N. Geschwind, A. Galaburda, M. Albert, and N. Gartrell. Towson, MD: The Orton Dyslexia Society.

Scanlon, D. M., and Vellutino, F. R. 1996. Prerequisite skills, early instruction, and success in first grade reading: Selected results from a longitudinal study. *Mental Retardation and Developmental Disabilities Research Review* 2:54–63.

Scarborough, H. S. 1989. Prediction of reading disability from familial and individual differences. *Journal of Educational Psychology* 81:101–8.

Scarborough, H.S. 1990. Very early language deficits in dyslexic children. *Child Development* 61:1728–43.

Scarborough, H. S. 1991a. Antecedents to reading disability: Preschool language development and literacy experiences of children from dyslexic families. *Reading and Writing* 3:219–33.

Scarborough, H. S. 1991b. Early syntactic development of dyslexic children. *Annals of Dyslexia* 41:207–20.

Scarborough, H. S. 1995, April. Long-term prediction of reading skills: Grade 2 to grade 8. Presented to the Society for Research in Child Development, Indianapolis.

Scarborough, H. S., and Dobrich, W. 1990. Development of children with early language delays. *Journal of Speech and Hearing Research* 33:70–83.

Scarborough, H. S., and Dobrich, W. 1994. On the efficacy of reading to preschoolers. *Developmental Review* 14:245–302.

Scarborough, H. S., Dobrich, W., and Hager, M. 1991. Preschool literacy experience and later reading achievement. *Journal of Learning Disabilities* 24:508–11.

Shapiro, B. K., Palmer, F. B., Antell, S., Bilker, S., Ross, A., and Capute, A. J. 1990. Precursors of reading delay: Neurodevelopmental milestones. *Pediatrics* 416–20.

Share, D. L., Jorm, A. F., Maclean, R., and Matthews, R. 1984. Sources of individual differences in reading acquisition. *Journal of Educational Psychology* 76(6):1309–24.

Shaywitz, S. E., Escobar, M. D., Shaywitz, B. A., Fletcher, J. and Makuch, B. 1992. Evidence that reading disability may represent the lower tail of a normal distribution of reading ability. *New England Journal of Medicine* 326:145–50.

Shaywitz, S. E., Shaywitz, B. A., Fletcher, J. M., and Escobar, M. D. 1990. Prevalence of reading disability in boys and girls. *Journal of the American Medical Association* 264:998–1002.

Snow, C. E., Tabors, P. O., Nicholson, P. A., and Kurland, B. F. 1995. SHELL: Oral language and early literacy skills in kindergarten and first grade children. *Journal of Research in Childhood Education* 10:37–48.

Spring, C., and Davis, J. M. 1988. Relations of digit naming speed with three components of reading. *Applied Psycholinguistics* 9:315–34.

Stanovich, K. E., Cunningham, A. E., and Cramer, B. R. 1984. Assessing phonological awareness in kindergarten children: Issues of task comparability. *Journal of Experimental Child Psychology* 38:175–90.

Stark, R., Bernstein, L., Condino, R., Bender, M., Tallal, P., and Catts, H. 1984. Four year follow-up study of language-impaired children. *Annals of Dyslexia* 34:49–68.

Stuart, M. 1995. Prediction and qualitative assessment of five- and six-year-old children's reading: A longitudinal study. *British Journal of Educational Psychology* 65:287–96.

Studdert-Kennedy, M., and Mody, M. 1995. Auditory temporal perception deficits in the reading-impaired: A critical review of the evidence. *Psychonomic Bulletin and Review* 2:805–14.

Tallal, P., and Stark, R. E. 1982. Perceptual motor profiles of reading impaired children with or without concomitant oral language deficits. *Annals of Dyslexia* 32:163–76.

Thomas, B. 1984. Early toy preferences of four-year-old readers and nonreaders. *Child Development* 55: 424–30.

Torgesen, J. In press. The prevention and remediation of reading disabilities: Evaluating what we know from research. *Academic Language Therapy.*

Tunmer, W. E., Herriman, M. L. and Nesdale, A. R. 1988. Metalinguistic abilities and beginning reading. *Reading Research Quarterly* 23:134–58.

Vellutino, F. R., and Scanlon, D. M. 1987. Phonological coding, phonological awareness, and reading ability: Evidence from a longitudinal and experimental study. *Merrill-Palmer Quarterly* 33(3):321–63.

Wagner, R. K., Torgesen, J. K., and Rashotte, C. A. 1994. Development of reading-related phonological processing abilities: New evidence of bidirectional causality from a latent variable longitudinal study. *Developmental Psychology* 30(1):73–87.

Walberg, H. J. and Tsai, S. 1985. Correlates of reading achievement and attitude: A national assessment study. *Journal of Educational Research* 78:159–67.

Walker, D., Greenwood, C., Hart, B., and Carta, J. 1994. Prediction of school outcomes based on early language production and socioeconomic factors. *Child Development* 65:606–21.

Watson, B. U., and Miller, T. K. 1993. Auditory perception, phonological processing and reading ability/disability. *Journal of Speech and Hearing Research* 36:850–63.

Weller, L. D., Schnittjer, C. J., and Tuter, B. A. 1992. Predicting achievement in grades three through ten using the Metropolitan Readiness Test. *Journal of Research in Childhood Education* 6:121–29.

Wells, G. 1985. Preschool literacy-related activities and success in school. In *Literacy, Language, and Learning*, eds. D. R. Olson, N. Torrance, and A. Hildyard. Cambridge: Cambridge University Press.

Wells, G., Barnes, S., and Wells, J. 1984. *Linguistic Influences on Educational Attainment.* Final Report to the Department of Education and Science.

White, K. R. 1982. The relation between socioeconomic status and academic achievement. *Psychological Bulletin* 91:461–81.

Wimmer, H., Landerl, K., Linortner, R., and Hummer, P. 1991. The relationship of phonemic awareness to reading acquisition: More consequence than precondition but still important. *Cognition* 40:219–49.

Wolf, M. 1991. Naming speed and reading: The contribution of the cognitive neurosciences. *Reading Research Quarterly* 26:123–41.

Wolf, M. in press. A provisional, integrative account of phonological and naming-speed deficits in dyslexia: Implications for diagnosis and intervention. In *Cognitive and Linguistic Foundations of Reading Acquisition: Implications for Intervention Research*, ed. B. Blachman. Hillsdale, NJ: Lawrence Erlbaum Associates.

Wolf, M., Bally, H., and Morris, R. 1986. Automaticity, retrieval processes, and reading: A longitudinal study in average and impaired readers. *Child Development* 57:988–1000.

Wolf, M., and Goodglass, H. 1986. Dyslexia, dysnomia, and lexical retrieval. *Brain and Language* 27:360–79.

Wolf, M., and Obregon, M. 1991. Early naming deficits, developmental dyslexia, and a specific deficit hypothesis. *Brain and Language* 42:219–47.

Wright, S., Fields, H., and Newman, S. 1991, August. On dyslexic classifications at age eight and thirteen. Presented to the 18th Scientific Conference of the Rodin Remediation Academy, Berne, Switzerland.

Zucker, S., and Riordan, J. 1990. One year predictive validity of new and revised conceptual language measurement. *Journal of Psychoeducational Assessment* 8:4–8.

APPENDIX

Table A-1. Prediction of Future Reading Achievement from Measures of Literacy Knowledge and Skills at About the Time of School Entry.

Study	N	Concepts of Print	Letter-Sound and Reading Skills	Combined	Letter Identi-fication Alone
Badian (1982)	143				.57
Badian (1994)	118				.52
Badian (1995)	81				.44
Blatchford et al. (1987)	343	.27			.61
Bowey (1995)	116				.60
Busch (1980)	1052		.56		.47
Butler et al. (1985)	320				.57
Chew and Lang (1990)	110				.49
Elbro et al. (1996)	91	.30			.69
Flynn and Flynn (1978)	81		.34		
Glazzard (1977)	87		.85		
Grogan (1995)	51		.45		
Gullo et al. (1984)	77		.57		
Horn and O'Donnell (1984)	218				.59
Juel et al. (1986)	80		.73		
Lundberg et al. (1980)	133		.64		
Mann (1984)	44				.52
Mann and Ditunno (1990)					
sample 1	31		.56		
sample 2	39		.51		
sample 3	32		.36		
Mason (1992)	109		.54		
McCormick et al. (1994)	38		.60		.52
Muehl and Di Nello (1976)	56				.41
Randel et al. (1977)	625		.51		
Rubin et al. (1978)	520		.62		
Scanlon and Vellutino (1996)	1000	.27	.64		.59
Scarborough (1989)	66		.36		
Share et al. (1984)	500				.63
Snow et al. (1995)	63	.54		.66	
Stanovich et al. (1984)	31		.52		
Stuart (1995)	30	.49	.75	.80	.76
Tunmer et al. (1988)	100	.50			.53
Vellutino & Scanlon (1987)					
sample 1	150		.44		.33
sample 2	61		.62		.66
sample 3	92		.53		.44
Wagner et al. (1994)	244			.51	
Weller et al. (1992)	415		.64		

			Type of Measure		
Study	N	Concepts of Print	Letter-Sound and Reading Skills	Combined	Letter Identi-fication Alone
Wells et al. (1984)	32	.82			
Wimmer et al. (1991)					
sample 1	50				.20
sample 2	42				.15
sample 3	36				.69
# of samples		7	22	2	24
median *r*		.49	.56	.73	.53
mean *r*		.46	.56	.73	.52
(*SD*)		(.20)	(.13)	n.a.	(.14)

Table A-2. Prediction of Reading Achievement from Phonological Awareness, Speech Discrimination, and Speech Production Abilities

Study	N	Phonological Awareness	Speech Discrimination	Speech Production
Badian (1995)	81	.42		
Bishop and Adams (1990)	76			.31
Bowey (1995)	116	.40		
Bradley and Bryant (1983)				
sample 1	118	.55		
sample 2	285	.46		
Bryant et al. (1990)	65	.66		
Busch (1980)	1052		.23	
Catts (1993)	56	.50		≤.26
Colarusso et al. (1980)	40		.19	
Elbro et al. (1996)	91	.33		.25
Felton (1992)	221	.33		
Grogan (1995)	51		.24	
Helfgott (1976)	31	.72		
Horn and O'Donnell (1984)	218		.28	
Hurford et al. (1993, 1994)	171	.40	.34	
Juel et al. (1986)	80	.60		
Levy and Stewart (1991)	56	.37		
Lundberg et al. (1980)	133	.43		
Mann (1984)	44	.75		
Mann and Ditunno (1990)				
sample 1	31		.02	
sample 2	39		.11	
sample 3	32		.16	
Muehl and Di Nello (1976)	56		.33	
Perfetti et al. (1987)	82	.42		
Scarborough (1989)	66	.38	.23	.19
Scanlon and Vellutino (1996)	1000	.42		
Share et al. (1984)	500	.64	.24	
Snow et al. (1995)	63	.58		
Stanovich et al. (1984)	31	.38		
Stuart (1995)	30	.34		
Tunmer et al. (1988)	100	.32		
Vellutino and Scanlon (1987)	126	.29		
Wagner et al. (1994)	244	.42		
Wimmer et al. (1991)				
sample 1	50	.45		
sample 2	42	.30		
sample 3	36	.60		
# of samples		27	11	4
median r		.42	.23	≤ .25
mean r		.46	.22	n.a.
(SD)		(.16)	(.09)	n.a.

Table A-3. Prediction of Reading Achievement from IQ Scores.

Study	N	Full-Scale	Verbal	Performance
Badian (1994)	118		.42	
Blatchford et al. (1987)	343		.36	
Bowey (1995)	116			.39
Bryant et al. (1990)	65	.68		
Busch (1980)	1052	.58		
Colarusso et al. (1980)	40		.25	
Elbro et al. (1996)	91			.22
Feshbach et al. (1977)				
sample 1		.39		
sample 2		.45		
Flynn and Flynn (1978)	81		.13	
Gullo et al. (1984)	77	.37		
Horn and O'Donnell (1984)	218		.51	
Lundberg et al. (1980)	133			.21
Mann & Ditunno (1990)				
sample 1	31	.52		
sample 2	39	.32		
sample 3	32	.31		
Mason (1992)	109		.50	
Massoth and Levenson (1982)	33	.33	.25	.38
Muehl and DiNello (1976)	56		.36	.35
Scanlon and Vellutino (1996)	1000		.38	.26
Scarborough (1989)	66	.31		
Stanovich et al. (1984)	31	.25		
Vellutino and Scanlon (1987)				
sample 1	150		.37	
sample 2	61		.41	
sample 3	92		.48	
Wimmer et al. (1991)				
sample 1	50			.24
sample 2	42			.04
# of samples		11	12	8
median r		.37	.38	.25
mean r		.41	.37	.26
(SD)	(.13)	(.11)	(.11)	

Table A-4.   Prediction of Reading Achievement from Lexical (Vocabulary) Skills

Study	N	Receptive Vocabulary	Expressive (Naming) Vocabulary	Rapid Serial Naming Colors, Objects	Digits, Letters
Badian (1982)	129		.36		
Badian (1994)	118		.49	.41	
Bishop and Adams (1990)	76	.44	.51		
Bowey (1995)	116	.46			
Bradley and Bryant (1983)					
sample 1	118	.52			
sample 2	285	.42			
Bryant et al. (1990)	65	.43			
Catts (1993)	56			.51	
Colarusso et al. (1980)	49	.21			
Elbro et al. (1996)	91	.25		.43	
Felton (1992)	221			.31	.36
Flynn and Flynn (1978)	81	.00			
Hurford et al. (1993, 1994)	171	.36			
Levy and Stewart (1991)	56			.29	.35
Mann (1984)	44				.42
Mann and Ditunno (1990)					
sample 1	31				.39
sample 2	39				.25
sample 3	32				.33
McCormick et al. (1994)	38	.43			
Scanlon and Vellutino (1996)	1000	.28		.32	
Scarborough (1989)	66	.31	.49	.21	
Share et al. (1984)	500	.40		.42	
Snow et al. (1995)	63	.44			
Tunmer et al. (!988)	100	.15			
Vellutino and Scanlon (1987)	150	.25			
Wagner et al. (1994)	244				.50
Wells et al. (1984)	32	.60			
Wimmer et al. (1991)					
sample 2	42	.12			
Wolf, Bally, and Morris (1986)	83			.39	.66
Wolf and Goodglass (1986)	89	.03	.38		
Zucker and Riordan (1990)	75	.51			
# of samples		20	5	9	8
median *r*		.38	.49	.39	.38
mean *r*		.33	.45	.37	.41
(*SD*)		(.17)	(.07)	(.10)	(.12)

Table A-5. Prediction of Later Reading by Measures of Language Skills and Verbal Memory.

Study	N	Overall Language Index	Receptive Syntax/ Morphology	Receptive Semantic/ Unspecified	Expressive Language Skills	Memory: Words, Digits	Memory: Stories, Sentences
Badian (1982)	143		.42	.25	.40		.52
Badian (1994)	118				.25		.27
Bishop and Adams (1990)*	76		.51	.41	.54		.52
Bowey (1995)	116		.35			.56, .25**	
Bradley and Bryant (1983)							
sample 1	118					.40	
sample 2	285					.24	
Bryant et al. (1990)	65						.51
Butler et al. (1985)	320	.45	.44				
Catts (1993)*	56			.30		.41	
Colarusso et al. (1980)	40				.40		
Day and Day (1983)	56				.05		.57
Elbro et al. (1996)	91					.34	
Felton (1992)	221					-.14	
Grogan (1995)	51					.47	
Juel et al. (1988)	80			.34			
Klein (1980)	678		.40				.46
Levy and Stewart (1991)	56	.27		.08			
Lindquist (1982)	351	.49					
Lunzer et al. (1976)	184					.32	.25
Mann (1984)	44		≤.29			.56	
Mann and Ditunno (1990)							
sample 1	31					.26	
sample 2	39					.53	
sample 3	32					.21	

Study	N	Overall Language Index	Receptive Syntax/ Morphology	Receptive Semantic/ Unspecified	Expressive Language Skills	Memory: Words, Digits	Memory: Stories, Sentences
Mason (1992)	109				.23	.56	
Muehl and Di Nello (1976)	56					.27	
Scanlon and Vellutino (1996)	1000		.30	.05	.08	.33	.34
Scarborough (1989)	66		.18				
Share et al. (1984)	500		.43	.42	.37	.31**	.41
Snow et al. (1995)	63						
Vellutino and Scanlon (1987)							
sample 1	150			.13	.39		
sample 2	61			.08	.50		.49
sample 3	92			.06	.27		.58
Wagner et al. (1994)	244			.54		.33	
Wells et al. (1984)	32	.64					
Wimmer et al. (1991)	42					.05**	
# of samples		4	9	11	11	18	11
median r		.47	.38	.25	.37	.33	.49
mean r		.46	≤.37	.24	.32	.33	.45
(SD)		(.15)	n.a.	(.17)	(.16)	(.17)	(.12)

*These samples included many children with diagnosed language impairments.

**Task was Pseudoword Imitation rather than recall of word/digit lists.

Table A-6. Prediction of Future Reading Achievement from Measures of Visual and Motor Skills.

Sample	N	Visual Perception	Visual-Motor Integration	Visual Memory	Motor Skills
Badian (1994)	118		.17	.33	
Badian (1995)	81		.10		
Busch (1980)	1052		.38		
Butler et al. (1985)	320	.44			.32
Colarusso et al. (1980)	40	.20	.15		
Flynn and Flynn (1978)	81		.02		
Grogan (1995)	51			.40	
Horn and O'Donnell (1984)	218			.48	.18
Linquist (1982)	105				.26
Lundberg et al. (1980)	133	.19			
Lunzer (1976)	184			.47	
Mann and Ditunno (1990)					
sample 1	31			.18	
sample 2	39			.22	
sample 3	32			.19	
Massoth and Levinson (1982)	33				.35
McCormick et al. (1994)	38		.11		
Scanlon and Vellutino (1996)	1000	.26		.23	
Scarborough (1989)	66	.01			
Share et al. (1984)	500				.14
# of samples		5	6	8	5
median *r*		.20	.13	.28	.26
mean *r*		.22	.16	.31	.25
(*SD*)		(.15)	(.12)	(.12)	(.09)

Table A-7. Predicting Future Reading Achievement from Multiple Kindergarten Measures

Study	Grade (From-To)	Combined Predictors	N	R^2	% At Risk	% RD	% Correct	PPP	NPP	Sensitivity	Specificity
Badian (1982)	K-3	Letter Names									
		WISC-Info.									
		Sent. Mem.									
		Counting									
		Drawing	129	.55	16	10	92	57	99	92	92
Badian (1994)	K-1	Early Ach.									
		VIQ									
		SES									
		age	118	.60							
		Early Ach.									
		VIQ, SES, age									
		Letter Names									
		Letter Discrim.									
		RSN-Objects									
		Syll. Counting	118	.63	21	13	91	48	99	93	90
Butler et al. (1985)	K-3	Factor Scores:									
		Language-1									
		Language-2									
		Vis. Skills									
		Motor Skills									
		Rhythm									
		sex	320	.50	10	10	91	56	95	56	95

Study	Grade (From-To)	Combined Predictors	N	R²	% At Risk	% RD	% Correct	PPP	NPP	Sensitivity	Specificity
Felton (1992)	K-3	IQ RSN-letters PA (oddity)	215	.41	26	10	80	31	97	81	80
Horn and O'Donnell (1984)	K-1	Letter Names Vis. Discrim. Vis-Motor Write Name Verbal Mem. Attention Teacher Rating and others	218	—	8	10	93	55	97	71	95
Hurford et al. (1994)	1-2	Grade 1 Reading PA (Deletion) Phon. Discrim. PPVT	171	—	13	15	97	88	100	100	98
Lundberg et al. (1980)	K-1	PIQ Vis. Perc. PA (segment) PA (reverse) sex	133	.54	27	27	87	75	91	75	91

Study	Grade (From-To)	Combined Predictors	N	R^2	% At Risk	% RD	% Correct	PPP	NPP	Sensitivity	Specificity
Scanlon and Vellutino (1996)	K-1	Letter Names Word Recogn.	1000	.41							
		Letter Names Word Recog'n Number Names Counting/Math PA (segment) and 23 others	1000	.49							
Share et al. (1984)	K-1	Letter Names PA (segment) Sent. Memoryy Copy Letters sex	479	.63							
Wells et al. (1984)	K-1	Conc. Print Oral Lang.	31	.71							
Samples of Children with Early Language Impairment											
Bishop and Adams (1990)	K-2	PIQ Lang. Production Lang. Compreh. Speech Prod.	81	.50							
Catts (1991)	K-1	PA (Deletion) RSN-Objects	41	.50			83	77	89		

Study	Grade (From-To)	Combined Predictors	N	R^2	% At Risk	% RD	% Correct	PPP	NPP	Sensitivity	Specificity
Samples Containing Many Children with Family History of RD											
Elbro et al. (1996)	K-2	Letter Names PA (Deletion, PA (Match 1st Sound) Distinctiveness of Phonol. Repres'ns of Words Speech Prod.	90	—	19	26	84	76	89	57	94
Scarborough (1989)	K-2	Family History Confr. Naming Letter Names PA (Rhyme, Match 1st Sound) Let-Sound	62	.43	39	37	82	75	97	78	95

RD = Reading Disability; PA = Phonological Awareness; RSN = Rapid Serial Naming.

% At Risk = percentage of sample below chosen cutoff on combined predictor measures.

% RD = percentage of sample below chosen cutoff on outcome reading measure.

% Correct = percentage of sample whose outcome status (RD or not) was correctly predicted.

PPP = Positive Predictive Power: percentage of children designated as at risk who became RD.

NPP = Negative Predictive Power: percentage designated as not at risk who did not become RD.

Sensitivity = percentage of the RD children who had been correctly identified as at risk.

Specificity = percentage of the non-RD children who had been correctly identified as not at risk.

Section • III

Identification and Evaluation

Chapter • 6

The Discrepancy Formula
Its Use and Abuse

Linda S. Siegel

Dyslexia is a condition in which individuals, despite average or above average intelligence, have great difficulty learning to read. Dyslexia is a diagnosis by exclusion; dyslexics have average or above average IQ test scores and have had adequate instruction in reading, and do not have neurological problems or significant emotional disturbances that might be considered responsible for their difficulty in acquiring reading skills.

THE DISCREPANCY DEFINITION

The traditional definition of a dyslexic is an individual with a significant discrepancy between his or her IQ and reading scores, so that the reading score is significantly lower than would be predicted by the IQ. This is the discrepancy definition of dyslexia. In this traditional conceptualization, the group of children who have reading problems but who show no significant discrepancy between IQ and reading scores are called poor readers and are not considered dyslexic.

THE ROLE OF IQ

The discrepancy definition assumes the validity of the intelligence test (IQ) score. Recently, there has been much debate about the use of the IQ score (Fletcher 1992; Francis et al. 1990; Siegel 1988a, 1988b, 1989a, 1990a, 1990b; Stanovich 1991). It is often argued that we need IQ tests to measure the "potential" of a child. This type of argument implies that there is some entity, called IQ, that is real and that will tell us how far a child can progress, how much he or she can learn, and what we can expect of that child. Presumably, the IQ score is a measure of logical reasoning, problem solving, critical thinking, and whatever we mean by intelligence. This sounds quite reasonable until one examines the content of the IQ test. Intelligence tests consist of measures of factual knowledge including questions about geography and history, definitions of words, memory, fine-motor coordination, and fluency of expressive language. They do not measure reasoning or problem-solving skills. They measure, for the most part, what a child has learned, not what he or she is capable of doing in the future. It is obvious that these types of questions measure what a child has learned, not fundamental problem–solving or critical thinking skills.

Another assumption of the proponents for the use of IQ test scores is that intelligence can be measured in the same way as height or weight. However, height is a physical dimension that has a physical reality. Intelligence is not a physical dimension but is a construct. There is no yardstick for the real IQ. Independent observers with different rules would arrive at the same number, within a few millimetres, for the height of a person. Independent IQ tests often arrive at quite different numbers for the IQ of a particular individual. There is universal agreement among scientists on what constitutes a millimetre, centimetre, inch, or yard; however, there is a great deal of controversy about the nature of intelligence and how to measure it.

I have argued that IQ tests do not really measure intelligence or potential; the IQ tests measure specific and usually learned skills such as vocabulary and specific factual knowledge. I claim that IQ tests are not particularly adequate measures of skills such as problem solving, logical reasoning, and/or adaptation to the environment. I have made a case for the biased nature of the content of IQ tests and how performance on the test might be subject to specific knowledge of specific facts. I seem to have convinced some individuals (Baldwin and Vaughn 1989) so that now the claim is that IQ tests do not measure potential but "that IQ test results are environmentally influenced and, at best, reflect a momentary level of intellectual functioning" (Baldwin and Vaughn 1989, p. 513). I could not agree more. If this is the case, I am even more confused as to why we need IQ test scores at all. Baldwin and Vaughn argue that IQ tests are not perfect but that this is not sufficient reason for doing away with them. My argument is that they are very far from perfect.

In spite of the obvious problems with IQ tests, many seem unwilling to abandon them. One of the major reasons for the use of IQ scores, according to the proponents for their use, seems to be that we must control IQ, presumably to obtain a "true" measure of whether or not there is a reading disability. Let us consider the logic of this position. The claim is made that we need to have a measure of general cognitive ability as a "gold standard" to assess what the reading score really represents. For example, Baldwin and Vaughn (1989) appear to argue that if we abandon the IQ test, we need to replace it with some type of assessment of ability. The assumption of this position is that we need this gold standard to be used in the educational system in order to ascertain whether or not a learning disability exists.

Torgesen (1989) argues that we need IQ tests to ensure that differences between learning disabled and normally achieving groups are not primarily the result of differences in "general learning aptitude" which appears to mean learning potential. However, Siegel (1988) has reported that there were significant differences between the reading disabled and normally achieving children at each IQ level, but no significant differences among reading disabled children at each IQ level. Furthermore, these differences in whatever IQ tests measure do not seem to be sufficient to explain the differences in cognitive functioning between reading disabled and normally achieving children. Torgesen claims that we need IQ tests because we want to be certain that the differences in cognitive processing are "not the result of pervasive intellectual differences between groups." The data that I have reported clearly show that the differences between the normally achieving and reading disabled group are not due to differences in IQ. The normally achieving readers had higher scores on the phonological, language, and memory tasks than the reading disabled group at every level of IQ. In addition, there were no differences on the phonological, reading, spelling, language, and memory tasks among the reading disabled children at each IQ level. These data clearly show that differences in IQ scores are not related to reading performance or problems. I remain perplexed as to why these data are ignored by those who argue for the use of IQ tests.

As Torgesen (1989, p. 484) has written, "Thus, there are no easily defensible conventions about which aspects of 'intelligence' to control when selecting samples of children with LD." There is no way to decide and no evidence that one particular IQ score is better than any other. Stanovich has noted that there is a great deal of controversy about what constitutes measures of intelligence. The point is that the nature and content of the questions on the IQ test are arbitrary. As Stanovich has said, "Obvious to the ongoing debates, specialists in learning disabilities seem to have avoided the issue by adopting a variant of E. G. Boring's dictum and acting as if "intelligence is what The Psychological Corporation says it is!" (Stanovich 1991, p. 10).

IQ AND LEARNING DISABILITIES

For the purpose of argument, let us consider the proposition that IQ is a measure of general cognitive ability that provides a standard against which we can measure reading. The IQ tests measure functions such as vocabulary, specific knowledge, memory, fine motor coordination, and short and long–term memory. All of these are deficient in children with reading problems. Therefore, the IQ tests will reflect the difficulties that children have in these areas. Proponents for the use of IQ tests argue that children who have low scores on reading tests should not be considered reading disabled if they have low scores on IQ tests. This reasoning is the ultimate in circularity because the low scores on the IQ tests are a consequence, not a cause, of their reading disability.

Rather than dealing with difficulties that learning disabled children have on IQ tests in the areas of language, memory, and fine-motor coordination, Baldwin and Vaughn say that I am merely providing a "list of excuses for why children with learning disabilities do poorly on IQ tests." These so-called "excuses" are not excuses, but reasons, even if Baldwin and Vaughn choose not to recognize the problem. Simply stated, the reason that the IQ score may be an under-estimate of the potential of many learning disabled children is that these children have difficulty with the question on the IQ test because of their learning disability. It seems circular and even cruel to suggest that someone is not capable, or less capable of learning because the very learning disability that they have affects their memory, language, or fine-motor skills, and is responsible for a lower score on an IQ test.

It might be argued that some children who are reading disabled have higher scores on the IQ test than other reading disabled children. Therefore, if my point is that having a reading disability means that the IQ score is an underestimate of "general cognitive ability," it is reasonable to ask why some reading disabled children have higher scores than others. There are several points that are relevant here. The IQ test is a mixture of a variety of skills; the same score can be arrived at with different profiles; and there is a premium on the knowledge of specific facts and vocabulary. It is quite reasonable to assume that different children, particularly children of different social classes , have had different exposure to this material. In a recent paper, Tunmer (1989) summarizes the political and social class biases that are represented by IQ tests. These biases result in questions about the usefulness of IQ as a means of identifying discrepancies among the reading disabled.

One of the implications of using the IQ test is that the IQ score "predicts" reading achievement. Olson (1986) analyzes this relationship as follows:

> But, do tests of intelligence measure some underlying quality of mind and thereby explain intelligent performance? Or do they simply, as I prefer to say, sample a domain of competence, thereby providing a description of a range of cognitive competence but not an explanation of how or why such competence would arise? To focus this question more sharply, do tests of intelligence give access to some underlying quality of mind that would explain a person's performance on cognitive tasks, or do they merely sample that competence in such a way as to give an indication of levels of performance in an domain, but in no way explain that level of competence?
>
> In the simplest case, IQ predicts reading comprehension. But why? What are these tests measuring? A basic quality of the mind that makes learning to read easy? Or a sample of specialized use of language common to both tests of intelligence and tests of reading. If it is the first, the IQ test would explain the good or poor reading competence itself. In that case, it would provide a description of the poor reading but not an explanation for that level of reading competence. (p. 39)

One of the arguments of the proponents for the use of IQ test scores has been that IQ correlates with achievement. Therefore, as it is a predictor of achievement, it is "useful" according to Graham and Harris (1989). Even if the IQ score was the ultimate measure of general achievement, it only correlates very moderately with school achievement. The best estimates are that the correlation is approximately .50, accounting for, at best, 25% of the variance. Parental education level or income is also correlated with achievement. Therefore, it would be as logical to use parental income as the standard (Tunmer 1989). The use of parental income makes as much sense as the use of IQ. Of course, I am not seriously making this suggestion but if IQ is used because it correlates with achievement, why not use parental income or education by the same logic? Obviously, this type of suggestion is counter to our egalitarian philosophy, but the logic is clear. It is not clear why IQ should continue to be used.

IQ AND LD: A CASE OF BIAS

There is an additional problem in the use of IQ tests with children who have learning disabilities. It is a logical paradox to use IQ scores with learning disabled children because most of these children are deficient in one or more of the component skills that are part of these IQ tests; and, therefore, their scores on IQ tests will be an underestimate of their competence. It seems illogical to recognize that a child has deficient memory and/or language and/or fine-motor skills and then say that the child is less intelligent because he or she has these problems.

There is another source of bias in the use of IQ tests, specifically, IQ discrimination against individuals from the lower socioeconomic classes. Siegel and Himel (in press) found that there was a significant positive correlation (0.351) between the IQ scores of children and socioeconomic status (SES) of the parents. Furthermore, the dyslexic children had significantly higher SES scores than the poor readers. IQ is significantly correlated with socioeconomic status, presumably a measure, at least in part, of a child's environment. If IQ reflects the environment (at least partially), then children from more disadvantaged environments would be expected to achieve lower scores on IQ tests. Thus, children from disadvantaged backgrounds would be less likely to be classified as dyslexic, even though they may have very severe reading problems, and more likely to be classified as poor readers. In many educational situations, these children would be denied the remedial help they need.

The proponents for the use of the IQ test assume that IQ is a valid measure of intelligence. In contrast, I would like to argue that IQ is actually a measure of the type of knowledge that is dependent to a large, but unknown, degree on the environmental experiences of the child. Therefore, we would expect the dyslexics, who as a group, have higher IQ scores than the poor readers, to have higher SES scores.

MATTHEW EFFECTS

Another issue in assessing the validity of the discrepancy definition is the problem of the "Matthew effects" as described by Stanovich (1986). This influence of reading problems on IQ and other cognitive processes has been described as "the tendency of reading itself to cause further development in other, related cognitive abilities, [i.e. IQ] such that the rich get richer and the poor get poorer" (Stanovich 1988a, p. 21).

The Matthew effect refers to the bi-directional relationship between reading and cognitive development. Certain minimum cognitive capabilities must be present to begin reading, but once reading commences, the act of reading itself further develops these same cognitive capabilities. This relationship of mutual reinforcement is called the Matthew effect. This Matthew effect of a reciprocal relationship between reading and other cognitive skills is reflected in a general IQ test and, consequently, undermines the validity of using an IQ discrepancy based criterion. Children who read more gain the cognitive skills and information relevant to the IQ test and, consequently, attain higher IQ scores. Children with reading problems read less, and therefore, fail to gain the skills and information necessary for higher scores on the IQ test. Therefore, because of a mutually reinforcing relationship between reading and IQ, independence is not satisfied and the use of an IQ based discrepancy definition for dyslexia is invalid based on variables closely related to the reading process. Researchers of reading disabled individuals have found no differences between dyslexics and poor readers. (See Toth and Siegel 1994, for a detailed review.)

If the Matthew effect, as described by Stanovich is operating, it would be expected that, with increasing age, there would be a decline in IQ scores because vocabulary and knowledge increase as a result, at least in part, of experiences with print. If reading disabled children have less experience with print than children without reading problems, the chance to acquire new knowledge is reduced and IQ scores will fall. Stanovich reviews studies to show that IQ scores decrease over time for the reading disabled children. The existence of Matthew effects are particularly relevant to the discussion of the role of IQ in the measurement of reading disability because Matthew effects cast doubts on the validity of the IQ measure, particularly for children with reading and other learning problems.

Siegel and Himel (in press) found that: (1) the mean IQ scores were lower for the older dyslexic children, suggesting an effective decline with age; and (2) the ratio of poor readers to dyslexic children increased with age. The findings strongly suggest that the measured IQ of dyslexic children decreases with age, leading to a reclassification from dyslexic to poor readers using the discrepancy approach. The lack of reading experience of dyslexic individuals, because they are less likely to read and, therefore, less likely to acquire new vocabulary and information, showed a drop in IQ scores with increasing age.

DYSLEXICS VERSUS POOR READERS: IS THERE A DIFFERENCE?

An assumption of the discrepancy definition is that children who are *dyslexic* and who have a discrepancy between their reading and IQ scores are different from those children who are *poor readers* and who have lower IQ scores and no discrepancy between reading and IQ. I have studied the differences between dyslexics and poor readers on a variety of phonological processing, language, and memory tasks (Siegel 1992). Although dyslexics had significantly higher IQ scores than the poor readers, these two groups did not differ in their performances on reading, spelling, phonological processing, and on most of the language and memory tasks. There were also no differences in reading comprehension between dyslexics and poor readers. In all cases, performances of *both* reading disabled groups were significantly below that of normal readers.

Reading disabled children, whether or not their reading is significantly below the levels predicted by their IQ scores, have significant problems in phonological processing, short-term and working memory, and syntactic awareness. On the basis of these data, there does not seem to be a need to differentiate between dyslexics and poor readers. Both of these groups are *reading disabled* and have deficits in phonological processing, verbal memory, and syntactic awareness. There does not appear to be any empirical evidence to justify distinctions between dyslexics and poor readers.

REMEDIATION

It might be argued that we need to use IQ test scores in the assessment of learning disabilities because IQ scores help us determine who would benefit from remediation. Presumably, children with higher IQ scores would be able to benefit more from educational experiences. In fact, the studies that have actually *measured* the relation between IQ and the effects of remediation have found that *learning disabled children with lower scores showed similar gains from remediation as did those with higher IQ scores* (Arnold, Smeltzer, and Barneby 1981; Kershner 1990; Lytton 1967; van der Wissel and Zegers 1985). Torgesen, Dahlem, and Greenstein (1987) found that, in some cases, gains in reading performance among reading disabled children were not related to IQ scores; but in others there was a small but statistically significant relationship. One study (Yule 1973) even found that "reading backward" children (poor readers) with lower IQ scores made *more* gains than "specifically reading disabled" children with higher IQ scores (dyslexics).

ASSESSMENT OF DYSLEXIA

These data suggest that the assessment of learning disabilities should concentrate on specific academic skills rather than on IQ scores. For diagnosing reading disability, the most appropriate measure appears to be, simply, a low reading score. These findings suggest that there is no need to use IQ tests to determine who is learning disabled.

The solution that I propose is to use achievement test scores and not an IQ achievement discrepancy to define a reading disability. Various aspects of the rationale for this decision are outlined in Siegel (1991) and Siegel and Heaven (1986). I propose that if an individual has a low score on a reading test, then that individual should be called reading disabled. Of course, certain other criteria, called exclusionary criteria, need to be applied, such as severe emotional problems, neurological deficits, inadequate educational opportunity, or insufficient knowledge of the language.

A test of word recognition is critical for the assessment of learning disabilities. Specifically, an assessment of a child with the possibility of a reading disability should include a measure of word recognition skills. These word recognition skills are the basis for gaining meaning from print and it is important to know if skills in this area are significantly below average. Furthermore, Stanovich (1986) and others, including my colleagues and I (Siegel 1986; Siegel and Ryan 1988, 1989b), have argued that phonological processing deficits, not low intellectual ability, are the core problems in cases of a reading disability. There is extensive evidence to support this point. (See Siegel 1993; Stanovich, 1988a, 1988b, for reviews.) One of the ways of assessing these skills involves reading pseudowords. Pseudowords are pronounceable combinations of English letters that can be sounded out using basic rules of phonics. This type of test assesses phonics, which is the key to decoding print in an alphabetic language such as English.

CONCLUSION

A reading disability, also called dyslexia, can be identified by standardized word recognition and pseudoword reading tests. A low score on these tests, compared to children of the same chronological age, constitutes a reading problem. There does not need to be a discrepancy between reading and an IQ score. Any child who displays severe problems with reading should receive remediation addressed to this problem. In conclusion, the IQ-achievement discrepancy scores serve no useful purpose in defining or understanding reading disabilities. It would be more helpful for children with reading disabilities if we concentrated on assessing and analyzing reading, spelling, arithmetic, and writing and providing appropriate remediation strategies for these problems.

REFERENCES

Arnold, L. E., Smeltzer, D. J., and Barneby, N. S. 1981. Specific perceptual remediation: Effects related to sex, IQ and parents' occupational status; behavioral change pattern by scale factors; and mechanisms of benefit hypothesis tested. *Psychological Reports* 49:198.

Baldwin, R. S., and Vaughn, S. 1989. Why Siegel's arguments are irrelevant to the definition of learning disabilities. *Journal of Learning Disabilities* 22:513–20.

Bell, L., and Perfetti, C. A. 1989. Reading ability, "reading disability" and garden variety low reading skill: Some adult comparisons. Unpublished manuscript.

Biemiller, A., and Siegel, L. S. 1997. A longitudinal study of the effects of the *Bridge* Reading Program for children at risk for reading failure. *Learning Disabilities Quarterly* 20:83–92.

Bloom, A., Wagner, M., Reskin, L., and Bergman, A. 1980. A comparison of intellectually delayed and primary reading disabled children on measures of intelligence and achievement. *Journal of Clinical Psychology* 36:788–90.

Cobrinik, L. 1974. Unusual reading disability in severely disturbed children. *Journal of Autism and Childhood Schizophrenia* 4:163–75.

Das, J. P., Mensink, D., and Mishra, R. K. 1990. Cognitive processes separating good and poor readers when IQ is covaried. *Learning and Individual Differences* 2:423–36.

Ellis, N., and Large, B. 1987. The development of reading. As you seek so shall you find. *British Journal of Psychology* 78:1–28.

Fischer, F. W., Liberman, I. Y., and Shankweiler, D. 1977. Reading reversals and developmental dyslexia: A further study. *Cortex* 14:496–510.

Fletcher, J. M. 1992. The validity of distinguishing children with language and learning disabilities according to discrepancies with IQ: Introduction to the special series. *Journal of Learning Disabilities* 25:546–48.

Francis, D. J., Espy, K. A., Rourke, B. A., and Fletcher, J. M. 1990. Validity of intelligence scores in the definition of learning disability: A critical analysis. In *Neuropsychological Validation of Learning Disability Subtypes*, ed. B. P. Rourke. New York: Guilford.

Friedman, G., and Stevenson, J. 1988. Reading processes in specific reading retarded and reading backward 13 year olds. *British Journal of Developmental Psychology* 6:97–108.

Graham, S., and Harris, K. R. 1989. The relevance of IQ on the determination of leaning disabilities: Abandoning scores as decision makers. *Journal of Learning Disabilities* 22:500–503.

Hall, J. W., Wilson, K. P., Humphreys, M. S., Tinzmann, M. B., and Bowyer, P. M. 1983. Phonetic similarity effects in good vs. poor readers. *Memory and Cognition* 11:520–27.

Johnston, R. S., Rugg, M. D., and Scott, T. 1987b. Phonological similarity effects, memory span and developmental reading disorders: The nature of the relationship. *British Journal of Psychology* 78:205–11.

Johnston, R. S., Rugg, M. D., and Scott, T. 1987a. The influence of phonology on good and poor readers when reading for meaning. *Journal of Memory and Language* 26:57–68.

Johnston, R. S., Rugg, M. D., and Scott, T. 1988. Pseudohomophone effects in 8 and 11 year old good and poor readers. *Journal of Research in Reading* 11:110–32.

Jorm, A., Share, D. L., Matthews, R. J., and Maclean, R. 1986. Behaviour problems in specific reading retarded and general reading backward children: A longitudinal study. *Journal of Child Psychology and Psychiatry* 27:33–43.

Kershner, J. R. 1990. Self-concept and IQ as predictors of remedial success in children with learning disabilities. *Journal of Learning Disabilities* 23:368–74.

Liberman, I. Y., Shankweiler, D., Orlando, C., Harris, K. S., and Berti, F. B. 1971. Letter confusions and reversals of sequence in the beginning reader: Implications for Orton's theory of developmental dyslexia. *Cortex* 7:127–42.

Lytton, H. 1967. Follow up of an experiment in selection of remedial education. *British Journal of Educational Psychology* 37:1–9.

Merrell, K. W. 1990. Differentiating low achieving students and students with learning disabilities: An examination of performances on the Woodcock-Johnson Psycho-Educational Battery. *The Journal of Special Education* 24: 296–305.

Olson, D. R. 1986. Intelligence and literacy: The relationships between intelligence and the technologies of representation and communication. In *Practical Intelligence*, ed. R. J. Sternberg and R. K. Wagner. Cambridge: Cambridge University Press.

Rack, J. P. 1989. Reading-IQ discrepancies and the phonological deficit in reading disability. Paper presented at the biennial meeting of Society for Research in Child Development, in April in Kansas City, MO.

Saloner, M. R., and Gettinger, M. 1985. Social interference skills in learning disabled and nondisabled children. *Psychology in the Schools* 2:201–7.

Scarborough, H. S. 1989a. A comparison of methods for identifying reading disabilities in adults. Unpublished manuscript.

Scarborough, H. S. 1989b. Prediction of reading disability from familial and individual differences. *Journal of Educational Psychology* 81:101–8.

Seidenberg, M. S., Bruck, M., Fornarolo, G., and Backman, J. 1985. Word recognition processes of poor and disabled readers: Do they necessarily differ? *Applied Psycholinguistics* 6:161–80.

Share, D. L., Jorm, A. F., McGee, R., Silva, P. A., Maclean, R., Matthews, R., and Williams, S. 1987. Dyslexia and other myths. Unpublished manuscript.

Siegel, L. S. 1984. A longitudinal study of a hyperlexic child: Hyperlexia as a language disorder. *Neuropsychologia* 22:577–85.

Siegel, L. S. 1986. Phonological deficits in children with a reading disability. *Canadian Journal of Special Education* 2:45–54.

Siegel, L. S. 1988a. Evidence that IQ scores are irrelevant to the definition and analysis of reading disability. *Canadian Journal of Psychology* 42:202–15.

Siegel, L. S. 1988b. Definitional and theoretical issues and research on learning disabilities. *Journal of Learning Disabilities* 21:264–66.

Siegel, L. S. 1989a. IQ is irrelevant to the definition of learning disabilities. *Journal of Learning Disabilities* 22:469–78, 486.

Siegel, L. S. 1989b. Why we do not need IQ test scores in the definition and analyses of learning disability. *Journal of Learning Disabilities* 22:514–18.

Siegel, L. S. 1990a. IQ and learning disabilities. R.I.P. In *Learning Disabilities: Theoretical and Research Issues*, eds. H. L. Swanson and B. Keogh. Hillsdale, NJ: Lawrence Erlbaum Associates.

Siegel, L. S. 1990b. Siegel's reply. [Letter to the editor]. *Journal of Learning Disabilities* 23:268–69, 319.

Siegel, L. S. 1991. Phonological processing, working memory, and syntactic awareness as determinants of reading skill. Paper presented at the International Conference on Memory in July in Lancaster, UK.

Siegel, L. S. 1991. The identification of learning disabilities: Issues in psycho-educational assessment. *Education and Law Journal* 3:301–13.

Siegel, L. S. 1992. An evaluation of the discrepancy definition of dyslexia. *Journal of Learning Disabilities* 25:618–29.

Siegel, L. S. 1993. Phonological pressing deficits as the basis of a reading disability. *Developmental Review* 13:246–57.

Siegel, L. S. 1994. The modularity of reading and spelling: Evidence from Hyperlexia. In *Handbook of Spelling: Theory, Process and Intervention*, eds. G. D. A. Brown and N. C. Ellis. Sussex, U.K.: John Wiley.

Siegel, L. S., and Heaven, R. K. 1986. Categorization of learning disabilities. In *Handbook of Cognitive, Social and Neuropsychological Aspects of Learning Disabilities*, Vol. 2, ed. S. J. Ceci. Hillsdale, NJ: Lawrence Erlbaum Associates.

Siegel, L. S., and Ryan, E. B. 1988. Development of grammatical sensitivity, phonological, and short-term memory skills in normally achieving and learning disabled children. *Developmental Psychology* 24:28–37.

Siegel, L. S., and Ryan, E. B. 1989a. The development of working memory in normally achieving and subtypes of learning disabled children. *Child Development* 60:973–80.

Siegel, L. S., and Ryan, E. B. 1989b. Subtypes of developmental dyslexia: The influence of definitional variables. *Reading and Writing: An Interdisciplinary Journal* 1:257–87.

Siegel, L. S. , and Himel, N. (in press). Socioeconomic status, age, and the classification of dyslexic and poor readers: The dangers of using IQ scores in the definition of reading disability. *Dyslexia*

Silva, P. A., McGee, R., and Williams, S. 1985. Some characteristics of 9-year-old boys with general reading backwardness or specific reading retardation. *Journal of Child Psychology and Psychiatry* 26:407–21.

Stanovich, K. E. 1986. Matthew effects in reading: Some consequences of individual differences in the acquisition of literacy. *Reading Research Quarterly* 21:360–407.

Stanovich, K. E. 1988a. Explaining the differences between the dyslexic and garden variety poor reader: The phonological-core variance-difference model. *Journal of Learning Disabilities* 21:590–604, 612.

Stanovich, K. E. 1988b. The right and wrong places to look for the cognitive locus of reading disability. *Annals of Dyslexia* 38:154–77.

Stanovich, K. E. 1991. Discrepancy definitions of reading disability: Has intelligence led us astray. *Reading Research Quarterly* 26:1–29.

Tal, N. F., Siegel, L. S., and Maraun, M. 1994. Reading comprehension: The role of question type and reading ability. *Reading and Writing: An Interdisciplinary Journal* 6:387–402.

Taylor, H. G., Satz, P., and Friel, J. 1979. Developmental dyslexia in relation to other childhood reading disorders: Significance and clinical utility. *Reading Research Quarterly* 15:84–101.

Torgesen, J. K. 1989. Why IQ is relevant to the definition of learning disabilities. *Journal of Learning Disabilities* 22:484–86.

Torgesen, J. K, Dahlem, W. E., and Greenstein, J. 1987. Using verbatim text recordings to enhance reading comprehension in learning disabled adolescents. *Learning Disabilities Focus* 3:30–38.

Toth, G., and Siegel, L. S. 1994. A critical evaluation of the IQ-achievement discrepancy based definition of dyslexia. In *Current Directions in Dyslexia Research*, ed. K. P. van den Bos, L. S. Siegel, D. J. Bakker, and D. L. Share. Liesse, The Netherlands: Swets and Zeitlinger.

Tunmer, W. 1989. Mental test differences as Matthew effects in literacy: The rich get richer and the poor get poorer. *New Zealand Sociology* 4:64–84.

van der Wissel, A., and Zegers, F. E. 1985. Reading retardation revised. *British Journal of Developmental Psychology* 3:3–9.

Yule, W. 1973. Differential prognosis of reading backwardness and specific reading retardation. *British Journal of Educational Psychology* 43:244–48.

This article was prepared with the assistance of a grant from the Natural Sciences and Engineering Research Council of Canada and while the author held a Killam Research Fellowship. The author wishes to thank Kim Kozuki for secretarial assistance.

Chapter • 7

Dyslexia *The Identification Process*

Doris J. Johnson

An evaluation to determine whether a person has dyslexia depends, in part, upon definitions of both dyslexia and reading. It also depends upon the goals of the evaluation—that is, whether testing is done primarily for classification and/or whether it is done to plan intervention. The latter is typically more extensive because many standardized tests yield only age or grade level information. Few, if any, provide sufficient data to determine whether students can apply phonics rules, can read various classes of words, or various types of texts. Therefore, a combination of both norm reference tests and criterion measures may be needed.

Over the years, and even today, dyslexia is defined in various ways. Often it is defined broadly as a reading disability that is not due to intellectual, sensory, motivational, or environmental factors, but is of constitutional origin. This type of definition emerged because, at one time, many reading problems were thought to be due primarily to emotional factors or lack of intelligence. However, several professionals have criticized such definitions because they focus on exclusionary, rather than inclusionary, criteria and because they are too broad (Rutter 1978; Lyon 1995). Recently, dyslexia has been defined by some professional groups as a problem with word recognition in order to differentiate it from more global language problems that are related to comprehension. Several theorists argue that decoding and comprehension are independent processes and that they should be differentiated for both research and diagnostic purposes. However, decoding problems usually interfere with acquisition of meaning.

The working definition of The Orton Dyslexia Society Research Committee from April, 1994 is provided below (Lyon 1995).

> Dyslexia is one of several distinct learning disabilities. It is a specific language-based disorder of constitutional origin characterized by difficulties in single word decoding, usually reflecting insufficient phonological processing. These difficulties in single word decoding are often unexpected in relation to age and other cognitive and academic abilities; they are not the result of generalized developmental disability or sensory impairment. Dyslexia is manifest by variable difficulty with different forms of language, often including, in addition to problems with reading, a conspicuous problem with acquiring proficiency in writing and spelling.

Lyon (1995) gave a clear rationale for each of the components. However, like other definitions of dyslexia and other handicapping conditions, the operationalization is usually more difficult than the definition per se. Diagnosticians still need to make decisions about levels of severity, types of tests, cut-off points, and many other factors. Furthermore, when planning for student needs, it is important to recognize that many problems co-occur. Some, but not all, dyslexic people have problems with oral syntax, morphology, and other aspects of language, reasoning, visual processing, and visual-motor integration, any one of which might interfere with reading or writing. Therefore, this chapter will include areas beyond work recognition that should be considered in an evaluation.

CASE HISTORY AND BACKGROUND INFORMATION

Information about the child's early development, language acquisition, health, and other factors is essential in any diagnostic study. Language delays or disorders are particularly important, as are indications of familial learning disabilities. Information about the literacy environments of children is also relevant. Diagnosticians should obtain information about the family background, primary and/or secondary languages, time spent reading in the home, and time spent reading to the child.

Data related to schooling, such as the nature of kindergarten programs and instructional approaches should be obtained. Some schools teach only letter sounds; thus, the children may do poorly when asked to say letter names rapidly. Others begin with whole language with little instruction on specific subskills. History of special services or tutoring is needed to know what types of approaches have been used. Thus, efforts are made to determine whether the child has profited from the instruction that has been provided.

PRELIMINARY STUDIES

Since many factors can contribute to reading disabilities, an evaluation should also include information regarding auditory and visual acuity, overall cognitive ability, and motivation. Tests for auditory and visual acuity are essential for determining whether a child has even mild impairments. Mild hearing losses or repeated ear infections can interfere with learning. Measures for visual acuity should be selected carefully because dyslexics with spatial orientation problems may have difficulty reading letter names and/or responding to E charts.

Information regarding overall cognitive ability is needed to differentiate children who may have general developmental delay from those who have a specific reading or learning disability. However, the types of measures may vary based on the theories of the investigator and the basic characteristics of the child. One would not measure the intelligence of a deaf student with a verbal intelligence test, nor that of physically handicapped person with tests that require perceptual motor skills. And, clearly, one would not use a group IQ test that required reading to assess dyslexic people even though such practices were not uncommon in the past.

At the present time, many school systems and diagnosticians determine whether a student is dyslexic or learning disabled by noting whether there is a discrepancy between intelligence and some reading measure. However, in recent years, many researchers and educators have opposed this practice and have raised questions about the relevance of IQ scores when making the diagnosis of reading disorder (Aaron 1991; Berninger et al. 1992). It is true that some children (e.g., hyperlexics) can decode words even though their intelligence scores are low. Conversely, some students are clearly dyslexic, but because various cognitive processing weaknesses interfere with the measurement of intelligence, they do not have a significant discrepancy between IQ and reading achievement.

While many questions have been raised regarding the use of a formula that requires a significant discrepancy between intelligence and achievement (Lyon 1995), information about cognitive ability is helpful in the diagnosis. Even if one does not accept the need for such a discrepancy, valuable information about verbal and visual-spatial-motor skills can be obtained from IQ tests, which can be used in the overall diagnosis and educational planning. For example, many studies of dyslexics have found low digit span and coding scores on the Wechsler Tests of Intelligence (1989, 1991). In an early study of sixty-five dyslexics, Johnson and Myklebust (1965) found that all subtest scores on the WISC were within normal limits, but that digit span was the lowest on the verbal scale. Intelligence tests may also yield information about a child's strengths. For example, some have excellent visual spatial skills. Others, despite low digit span scores, have remarkably good listening skills and are able to remember information they hear. Others have both listening and reading problems (Johnson 1994a). This information is important for recommending school accommodations and for determining whether students have reading comprehension problems beyond those related to poor word recognition (Olson et al. 1994). Problems related to speed of processing might also be identified on the Wechsler scales since all of the performance items are timed.

In a study of 21 six- and seven-year-olds, Johnson and Nummy (1996) reported that children with relatively global language disorders were usually identified by age three and that their verbal intelligence scores were lower than performance. In contrast, children who were later classified as primarily dyslexic had overall higher mental ability than those who had primary oral language problems, and were generally not identified until late kindergarten or early first grade.

In certain instances, because of possible cultural and experiential factors, diagnosticians use nonverbal intelligence tests such as the Leiter (Levine 1982), the Columbia (Burgemeister, Blum, and Lorge 1972), or the Test of Nonverbal Intelligence (Brown, Sherbenou, and Johnson 1990).

Intelligence test profiles may be useful in identifying possible subgroups, though we emphasize that a diagnosis of a learning or reading disability should never be made from an intelligence test. Achievement scores are essential. Certain children with nonverbal learning disabilities often have early reading problems that are different from those based primarily on phonological weaknesses (Johnson and Myklebust 1967; Rourke 1989). Such children often have high verbal and low performance scores on intelligence tests because of visual-spatial weaknesses. They perform poorly on tests of visual perception (Colarusso and Hammill 1972) and the visual portions of readiness tests. They, like other poor readers, have problems with word recognition; yet they perform well on rhyming and phonological awareness tests. With appropriate intervention during the early grades, many become successful readers, although some have higher-level listening and reading comprehension problems.

The ultimate goal of reading is comprehension; however, it is well known that many factors can interfere with the acquisition of meaning. As stated above, current definitions emphasize that dyslexic people usually have word recognition problems. An inability to recognize or decode words quickly interferes with meaning. In these cases, comprehension is a secondary problem. In contrast, some children have comprehension problems over and above their word recognition weaknesses. These may be related to co-occurring conceptual difficulties, oral language problems, and/or faulty, nonaccommodating reading strategies (Maria and MacGinitie 1982).

A LIFE SPAN PERSPECTIVE

Dyslexia and other learning disabilities can and do occur across all age ranges. Therefore, a developmental perspective is essential. In general, problems will not be identified until children have been exposed to certain content or taught certain skills. Concerns arise when children fail to profit from experience and/or when they fail to meet certain expectations. Thus, dyslexia will typically not be identified until children have been exposed to print, although those with histories of language problems, cognitive weaknesses, or familial disabilities may be considered at risk. Often the first concerns regarding reading arise in kindergarten or first grade. However, because many educators acknowledge wide variations in development, they may be reluctant to refer the child for further study. Nevertheless, considerable recent information regarding early predictors of reading difficulty should alert educators to the need for early intervention, particularly in the areas of oral language and phonemic awareness.

A life span perspective of reading development, presented by Chall in her book on Stages of Reading (1983), can be used in planning assessment and instruction. In her earliest stage, Chall emphasizes skills such as print awareness—reading logos, signs, or labels in the environment—and other forms of emergent literacy. At this stage, children should make predictions about word meaning from context and should be rhyming, playing with sounds, and telling stories, all of which contribute to literacy. In first grade, Chall emphasizes word recognition and early decoding. She says children cannot continue to guess from context. Somewhat later, children begin to read simple, familiar texts in order to develop fluency. At this stage, they use their background knowledge and are less tied to print. At the upper levels, students may need work on higher level decoding and word attack strategies, but the emphasis is more on comprehension, reasoning, and obtaining multiple perspectives of the world.

This life span perspective is useful in planning; however, dyslexic people may differ in several ways. First, they may have so much difficulty with work recognition and decoding that they do not attain any fluency. If they have good listening skills, they may achieve world views on many subjects, even though hey cannot acquire information from reading. Therefore, they may be at a low level stage in reading and at the upper level in listening. These uneven patters of development have been noted among college students with dyslexia. In order to master knowledge, they need to have people read to them or they need to be exceptional observers and listeners. Some may be lacking in knowledge if they have not been exposed to literature, social studies, or science via listening or observation. Needless to say, the demands for good auditory memory in these cases is great. Because listening comprehension is often good among dyslexic persons, some researchers recommend that the diagnosis be made by investigating discrepancies between listening comprehension and reading rather than discrepancies between intelligence and reading.

To illustrate the possible advantage of such an approach, we recently evaluated a nineteen-year-old who would not have met the criteria for dyslexia if a significant discrepancy between intelligence and word recognition scores were required (IQ 84; Reading SS 79, but he would have been classified, if a discrepancy between listening comprehension (SS 1015) and reading were accepted. His low digit span, coding, and arithmetic scores contributed to his relatively low intelligence. This case and many others raise both philosophical and theoretical questions about the criteria for classification. In particular, they raise issues regarding quantitative requirements and clinical judgment. In most cases, diagnosticians need to integrate test scores and observations.

The remainder of this chapter is devoted to areas that should be included in the assessment of reading and related areas of learning.

WORD RECOGNITION

The assessment of word recognition skills typically begins with a standardized test of oral reading such as the Wide Range Achievement Test (Wilkinson 1993), Letter-Word Identification from the Woodcock-Johnson (1989), or the Peabody Individual Achievement Test (Markwardt 1989). Typically, words in these tests are selected according to frequency of occurrence rather than specific patters or phonics rules. Olson et al. (1994) reported that some words in these tests are relatively regular while others are exceptions and, therefore, require sight word recognition. Standardized tests of this type are often problematic, particularly in the early grades. Because they have so few items at any age level, it is difficult to be certain what children know. While they provide some preliminary data, more criterion reference tests such as the Decoding Skills Test (Richardson 1985) or experimental measures such as those used by Olson et al. (1994) may be needed. These lists are designed to evaluate a student's ability to read several words with various syllable types (e.g., CVC; VCE) and words with two or more syllables. Johnson (1987) used various types of word lists including high imagery nouns, words with consistent letter/sound correspondence, familiar words with various morphological units, and word list from Shankweiler and Liberman (1972) that was designed to elicit single letter reversals (e.g., dig/big) and full word reversals (e.g., not/ton). I found that some dyslexic persons performed best when given high imagery nouns. Many had difficulty with words containing consonant blends. Some, but not all, reversed letters, but the reversals they made in reading were not the same as in spelling. In general, lists should be selected to address a question, e.g., "Can the child read words that have consistent letter/sound correspondence?" Words should also be appropriate for age and grade level. Without some concern for age level, easily decodable real words may actually be nonsense words for young children (e.g., din/kin). In severe cases, a full tabulation of all letter sounds the child knows, at the level of recognition and recall, may be needed.

Many researchers and teachers include measures of word attack (Woodcock-Johnson 1989) or reading of nonwords (e.g., aylerow) in the assessment. Such measures have been used for many years and have been found to discriminate dyslexic readers from other poor readers. Myklebust and Boshes (1969) reported that the Syllabication subtest from the Gates-McKillop (1962) was the best discriminator between a large group of third- and fourth-grade students with learning disabilities and a control group. An analysis of individual students, however, indicates that some people can read real words at an expected level, but not nonwords. In these cases, the diagnosis of dyslexia becomes somewhat questionable.

ORAL READING OF CONTEXT

Oral reading of passages and various types of text should be a part of the evaluation to further determine decoding, word recognition, and fluency skills. Studies have found that some children read certain words in context more accurately than in lists. This is especially evident on nonphonetic words such as "where, which, and there." If the content is familiar, some children read much better because they use their background knowledge and language. Even though such students may need work at the level of the word, they should have an opportunity to read texts to gain confidence and the sense that they can, indeed, read. Sometimes dyslexic children reported that they were not permitted to read texts until they achieved one hundred percent accuracy on syllables or word lists. As stated above, we recommend that they be given texts that allow them to use their background knowledge, and, if possible, obtain some fluency.

READING COMPREHENSION

Although current definitions of dyslexia tend to emphasize problems related to word recognition, all reading evaluations should include tests for comprehension of words and sentences, and various types of discourse including narratives, exposition, and even mathematics.

In choosing texts or tasks, diagnosticians should consider modes of responses that are required. Many group tests require a simple marking response such as matching words to pictures, or circling the correct answer. In contrast, some, such as The Passage Comprehension from the Woodcock-Johnson (1989) require the student to say a word that would best complete the text. Such tests require both comprehension and word retrieval. Thus, a student may do poorly for several reasons. Other tests require more complex verbal responses such as summaries. These may, in some cases, more accurately measure comprehension than recognition tasks, but if the student has verbal expression problems, they may not be valid measures of reading comprehension. Other tests require responses after the text is removed. These obviously have an additional memory component; and yet, they are real world tasks. Each of these formats places a different cognitive demand upon the child. Therefore, a comparison across tasks will yield useful diagnostic information. The ultimate goal is to determine how much of what type of information the student understands, with and without cued recall.

Reading comprehension should be compared with texts for reasoning and listening comprehension to try to determine the source of the weakness. In the early grades, listening comprehension typically exceeds reading comprehension, but after word recognition improves, reading comprehension is often better than listening because of the auditory memory demands on listening. Various patterns can be observed among students with learning disabilities.

ORAL LANGUAGE

Reading is often considered as a second order symbol because it is acquired after oral language. Therefore, reading evaluations should include assessments of both receptive and expressive language. Receptive language or listening comprehension is particularly important because failure to understand the primary language usually interferes with comprehension of other symbol systems. Furthermore, reading is a receptive form of language whereas writing is expressive.

Various processes within receptive language need to be investigated (Johnson 1994b) including discrimination, memory, and interpretation. Typically, receptive tasks should require little or no verbal output. Examples of tests that have receptive measures include Carrow-Woolfolk (1985), Dunn and Dunn (1981), German (1986), Goldman, Fristoe, and Woodcock (1970), Hresko, Reid, and Hammill (1991), Newcomer and Hammill (1982), Wiig and Secord (1989), and portions of the Woodcock-Johnson (1989).

Several components of expressive language should also be tested even though reading does not necessarily require any verbal output.

In recent years, several studies have indicated that poor readers have difficulty with rapid naming of figures or colors (Wolf 1984; Badian 1994). However, problems with picture naming were identified many years ago by Jansky and de Hirsch (1972). Tests for retrieval and picture naming are included in measures developed by Gardner (1990), German (1986), and others listed above. Other poor readers have difficulty with repetition of words and nonwords. These findings highlight difficulties with phonological coding.

Other investigators have found that poor readers also have difficulty with syntax (Siegel and Ryan 1984; Vogel 1975). Failure to acquire oral grammar interferes with the prediction and monitoring of text. Tests for sentence repetition (Carrow 1974), sentence memory, and sentence building, as well as spontaneous language samples, can be used to study grammar.

Formulation and organization problems interfere with understanding and/or summarizing material that has been read. Therefore, the ability to tell narratives can be included in the testing.

Because reading is a second order symbol system, children need to understand relationships between oral and written language, including the ways in which spoken words are represented in print (i.e., spacing, organization), prosody (at least partially represented with punctuation), and the relationships between phonology and orthography. In other words, linguistic awareness plays an important role in reading (Hook and Johnson 1978).

PHONOLOGICAL AWARENESS

In order to explore the possible reasons for poor word recognition, several subskills should be examined including phonological and orthographic awareness. The former is particularly critical. Many tasks have been developed for phonological awareness, including segmenting words by phonemes (Liberman 1973), sound categorization (Bryant and Bradley 1985), phoneme deletion, rhyming, and pig latin (Hook and Johnson 1978; Torgesen and Bryant 1994). Data from these tasks are powerful predictors of word recognition.

VISUAL PROCESSES

Although recent studies have identified phonological awareness as a core component of dyslexia, one cannot ignore the fact that reading requires the interpretation of visual symbols. Some dyslexic readers have problems with speed or visual processing demonstrated by low scores on Visual Matching (sets of numerals) and Cross-Out (geometric figures) on the Woodcock Johnson Psycho-educational Battery (1989). Johnson (1996) reported that a group of postsecondary students scored below expectancy on these tests, but that the performances varied according to their WAIS (Wechsler 1981) profiles. Those with significantly lower verbal intelligence scores than performance scores tended to perform better on Cross-Out, whereas those with opposite profiles performed better on Visual Matching. It was hypothesized that verbal mediation can be used on Visual Matching, that is students can say the numerals, but they cannot label the abstract geometric shapes. As indicated previously, dyslexic students often have low scores on the Coding subtest of the Wechsler (1991), but motor speed may also be a factor on this test.

Occasionally, young dyslexic students perform below expectancy on the Motor Free Test of Visual Perception (Colarusso and Hammill 1972); however, good performance does not necessarily mean a person is free from visual processing weaknesses, since many of the items are relatively simple and require only perception or memory of nonverbal figures. A careful analysis of the errors may reveal patterns that can be explored in more detail. For example, the test includes items for visual perception, spatial orientation, memory, figure ground, and closure.

Item analyses of the visual sections of reading readiness tests such as the Metropolitan (Nurss and McGauvran 1986) are also useful. Both single letter and word matching tasks are included. Several years ago Jansky and de Hirsch (1972) found that word matching was one of five measures that predicted reading achievement in second grade. More recently, Badian (1994) found that visual discrimination (orthographic) processing predicted reading achievement at the third-grade level.

Visual memory for letters and words should also be investigated because children are expected to retain images of letters and sight words. The information is needed not only to identify possible weaknesses, but to explore strengths and possible strategies for early reading. Studies have indicated that some dyslexic people can learn whole words and ideographic symbols. Although they cannot become efficient readers without learning to decode unfamiliar words, a tabulation of the logos and sight words they can read is helpful. Often, during remediation, work on decoding can proceed from the known to the unknown.

Revisualization of letters is essential for writing and should also be evaluated (Johnson and Myklebust 1967). Some children can copy but cannot access the visual image. In certain instances, they recall the visual pattern, but not the motor plan. Various procedures can be used to investigate revisualization. For example, one can ask students to first copy numerals and letters and then write from dictation to note possible discrepancies. However, they must know the letter names in order to write from dictation. We also use letter completion tasks and ask students to make specific letters (e.g., "Make this into an H, a B" or "Write any letters you know."). Occasionally, children with revisualization problems misspell words in writing that they can spell orally. Older students also tend to mix manuscript upper and lower case, and/or cursive letters because they cannot recall the visual image or motor patters for letters (Johnson and Blalock 1987).

ORTHOGRAPHIC AWARENESS

Dyslexic students may have few, if any, problems in visual discrimination or memory, but they frequently have problems with tasks that require more conscious awareness of the orthography and forms of representation. For example, some cannot read various type fonts and scripts. A second-grader said, "I can read words with the pointy letters." What he meant was that reading words in upper case was easier than lower case. He had a particularly difficult time with the multiple forms of A, a, a. To check for possible weaknesses, students are asked to match letters and words with various type fonts in both upper and lower case (BAT versus bat). If they have been exposed to cursive writing, they also match those forms with print. Many reading readiness and diagnostic tests include items of this type.

Part-to-whole relationships or the ability to identify the same patterns within words is also a relevant skill for reading. Some readiness tests (Nurss and McGauvran 1986), have a section in which children are asked to identify a pattern such as "an," in various positions within words (e.g., animal, planting, can). In some respects these tasks are comparable to phonological awareness tasks that require students to *listen* for similar patterns with words. Usually, however, the visual/orthographic tasks are easier because they do not require the auditory memory load of phonological awareness tasks.

PHONO-ORTHOGRAPHIC SKILLS

Reading requires the integration of spoken and written symbols. One cannot read with phonological skills alone, and not much with visual skills alone. Therefore, it is necessary to determine whether students know letter names, sounds, syllables, and words at the level of recognition and recall. Most group readiness tasks require recognition responses ("Mark s, /t/, ap, dog") whereas individual tests usually require oral responses. Both are important in order to find out what children know and what they can access. Many researchers have found that saying letter names is a good predictor of early reading (Jansky and de Hirsch 1972). Nevertheless, when planning interventions for people who have retrieval, articulation, or motor problems. it is helpful to use recognition or multiple choice responses ("Is this /m/ or /n/?") as well as recall. Speed of both recognition and recall should be investigated also.

The terminology in reading and reading disabilities varies considerably, along with labels for various tasks. Hence, a detailed description of each type of task is needed. For example, some phonological coding or awareness tasks require only oral skills (e.g., segmenting words by phonemes or blending). At other times, pictures may be used (e.g., "Mark the pictures that start with /m/."); and in still others, letters or printed words may be used. Obviously, the latter are much more closely related to reading and spelling and require more than phonological skills. Sometimes the reading of nonwords is classified as a phonological coding test, but in reality it requires both phonology and orthography. In the future it would be helpful if researchers and diagnosticians would clearly differentiate those tasks that do and do not require the integration of spoken and written symbols.

VISUAL-MOTOR SKILLS

Although reading does not require visual-motor output, the ability to copy and produce letters is typically needed for spelling unless severe motor handicaps necessitate the use of word processors and other devices. Often faulty handwriting is an indicator of a learning disability or neurological handicap. Johnson and Carlisle (1996) found a significant difference between a group of second-grade normally achieving and learning disabled children. Poor letter formation often contributes to an inability to read or monitor one's own work. Students in reading programs that require extensive writing may need alternative ways of responding in order to demonstrate their reading and spelling skills.

SPELLING

Writing and spelling frequently strengthen and stabilize the images of words. In addition, according to Bryant and Bradley (1980), spelling requires more analytical skills than reading. They theorize that reading requires visual chunking strategies whereas spelling requires more phonological, analytical strategies. They base this theory on the fact that some children spell certain words that they cannot read, particularly words that have relatively consistent letter-sound correspondence. For example, a child may write the word "must" correctly, but read it as "mut," or "mast," or "much." Although some components of reading typically precede writing, it is not unusual to see slightly higher spelling than reading scores among young elementary school children.

MATHEMATICAL SYMBOLS

Although the focus of this chapter is on reading, an evaluation of numerical symbols is helpful for both theoretical and educational purposes. With regard to theory, it is important to differentiate problems specific to one type of symbol (e.g., reading) from those that are more pervasive. If one seeks to identify specific reading disabilities, then one may wish to rule out all problems that interfere with symbols other than reading. However, many students with learning disabilities often have problems with more than one symbol system or area of achievement. Similarly, young children with language disorders frequently have problems with symbols such as gesture, pantomime, and pretend play. In a recent analysis of twenty-five six- to seven-year-olds, Johnson and Nummy (1996) reported that the majority, particularly those with oral language problems, were performing below expectancy in many areas of learning. The children with receptive language problems had difficulty with most symbol systems. In contrast, some dyslexic children, whose primary problems are related to word recognition, have fewer problems with symbols such as arithmetic, since numbers require less linguistic awareness. Such children do, of course, have difficulty reading story problems. On the other hand, some dyslexic students, particularly those with visual-spatial and visualization problems, have difficulty with both letter and numerals. For instance, and eight-year-old nonreader had problems with both letter and numeral recognition and with the production of both types of symbols.

Other symbol systems, such as music, may also require careful study. Researchers have found that some dyslexic people perform well on pure auditory music skills, but they cannot read music.

MOTIVATION AND AFFECTIVE FACTORS

Any investigation of learning problems needs to include information regarding motivation, goals, interests, and reactions to failure when a problem has already been identified. Although dyslexia is not due primarily to emotional factors, one cannot ignore the impact of failure and what it means to go to school daily without being able to read. As with any handicapping condition, the reactions and adjustments to problems vary from denial, to anger, disappointment, and finally acceptance. Often both the families and children go through several stages of reaction. Perhaps the most important goal is to maintain a sense of self respect and esteem even though certain skills or concepts are difficult to learn.

With regard to assessment, diagnosticians may use questionnaires, rating scales, or interviews to explore the child's attitudes toward learning, the perceptions about things that are easy or difficult, and general reactions to problems. When many negative feelings have been built up, it is often necessary to deal with those before formal instruction in reading can begin. In other cases, children are relieved when help is provided and when they see evidence of progress. Reactions to the time and place of intervention may also need to be considered. Some students dislike leaving the classroom, whereas others do not object. Some families prefer private intervention if they can afford it. In recent years, with the emphasis on collaboration in the classroom, more students are aware of the types of special services given for various handicapping conditions; so they feel less stigmatized when services are offered. Often, when helping students understand their problems and/or feeling about their problems, they can be given books about successful children and the ways in which the coped (Cicci 1995; Lauren 1997; Smith 1994).

DIAGNOSTIC TEACHING

Finally, in many instances, a few sessions of trial teaching adds significant information to the diagnostic process. Teachers can explore rate of learning responses to instruction and retention. Rather than acquiring a single "snapshot" from testing, one can gain a more realistic picture of the student's ability to profit from various types of instruction. Even though research has highlighted the word recognition problems of dyslexics, the individual patterns of strengths and weaknesses must always be considered.

REFERENCES

Aaron, P. G. 1991. Can reading disabilities be diagnosed without using intelligence tests? *Journal of Learning Disabilities* 24(3):178–86.

Badian, N. 1994. Preschool prediction: Orthographic and phonological skills and reading. *Annals of Dyslexia* 44:3–25.

Berninger, V., Hart, T., Abbott, R., and Karovsky, P. 1992. Defining reading and writing disabilities with and without IQ: A flexible, developmental perspective. *Learning Disability Quarterly* 15:103–18.

Bradley, L., and Bryant, P. 1985. *Rhyme and Reason in Reading and Spelling* (Monograph Series No. 1) Ann Arbor: University of Michigan Press/International Academy for Research in Learning Disabilities.

Brown, L., Sherbenou, R. J., and Johnson, S. K. 1990. *Test of Nonverbal Intelligence* 2nd ed. Austin, TX: PRO-ED.

Bryant, P., and Bradley, L. 1980. Why children sometimes write words which they cannot read. In *Cognitive Processes in Spelling*, ed. U. Frith. London: Academic Press.

Burgemeister, B. B., Blum, L. H., and Lorge, I. 1972. *Columbia Mental Maturity Scale*. New York: Harcourt, Brace, Jovanovich.

Carlisle, J., and Johnson, D. 1989. Assessment of school-age children. In *The Assessment of Learning Disabilities: Preschool Through Adulthood*, ed. L. Silver. Boston, MA: Grune & Stratton.

Carrow, E. 1974. *Elicited Language Inventory*. Austin, TX: Learning Concepts.

Carrow-Woolfolk, E. 1985. *Test for Auditory Comprehension of Language, rev. ed.* Allen, TX: DLM Teaching Resources.

Chall, J. 1983. *Stages of Reading Development*. New York: McGraw-Hill.

Cicci, R. 1995. *"What's Wrong with Me?" Learning Disabilities at Home and School*. Baltimore: York Press.

Colarusso, R. P., and Hammill, D. D. 1972. *Motor-Free Visual Perception Test*. Navato, CA: Academic Therapy Publications.

Dunn, L., and Dunn, L. 1981. *Peabody Picture Vocabulary Test-Revised*. Circle Pines, MN: American Guidance Service.

Gardner, M. F. 1990. *Expressive One-Word Picture Vocabulary Test-Revised*. Austin, TX: PRO-ED.

Gates, A., and McKillop, A. 1962. *Gates-McKillop Reading Diagnostic Test*. New York: Teachers College Press.

German, D. J. 1986. *Test of Word Finding*. Allen, TX: DLM Teaching Resources.

Goldman, R., Fristoe, M., and Woodcock, R. W. 1970. *Goldman-Fristoe, Woodcock Test of Auditory Discrimination*. Circle Pines, MN: American Guidance Service.

Hook, P., and Johnson, D. J. 1978. Linguistic awareness in proficient and disabled readers. *The Orton Society Bulletin* 28:62–78.

Hresko, W. P., Reid, D. K., and Hammill, D. D. 1991. *Test of Early Language Development*. 2nd ed. Austin, TX: PRO-ED.

Jansky, J., and de Hirsch, K. 1972. *Preventing Reading Failure*. New York: Harper & Row.

Johnson, D. 1987. Reading disabilities. In *Adults with Learning Disabilities*, eds. D. Johnson and J. Blalock. Orlando: Grune and Stratton.

Johnson, D. 1994a. Clinical study of adults with severe learning disabilities. *Learning Disabilities* 5(1):43–50.

Johnson, D. 1994b. Measurement of listening and speaking. In *Frames of Reference for the Assessment of Learning Disabilities*, ed. G. R. Lyon. Baltimore: Brookes.

Johnson, D. 1996. Patterns of problems among postsecondary students with learning disabilities. Paper presented to *The Orton Dyslexia Society*, Boston.

Johnson, D. J., and Myklebust, H. 1965. Dyslexia in childhood. In *Learning Disorders*, ed. J. Hellmuth. Seattle, WA: Special Child Publications.

Johnson, D., and Myklebust, H. 1967. *Learning Disabilities: Educational Principles and Practices*. New York: Grune & Stratton.

Johnson, D., and Blalock, J. (eds.). 1987. *Adults with Learning Disabilities*. Orlando, FL: Grune & Stratton.

Johnson D., and Carlisle, J. 1996. A study of handwriting in written stories of normal and learning disabled children. *Reading and Writing* 8(1):45–49.

Johnson, D. J., and Nummy, J. C. 1996. Learning disabilities in early childhood. Paper presented at Learning Disabilities Association Conference, Dallas, Texas.

Lauren, J. 1997. *Succeeding with L. D.* Minneapolis: Free Spirit Publishing.

Levine, M. N. 1982. *The Leiter International Performance Scale Handbook.* Los Angeles, CA: Western Psychological Services.

Levine, M. N. 1986. *The Leiter International Performance Scale.* Chicago, IL: Stoelting Company.

Liberman, I. 1973. Segmentation of the spoken words and reading acquisition. *Bulletin of The Orton Society* 23:65–77.

Lyon, G. R. 1995. Toward a definition of dyslexia. *Annals of Dyslexia* 45:3–27.

Maria, K., and MacGinitie, W. 1982. Reading comprehension disabilities: Knowledge structures and non-accommodating text processing strategies *Annals of Dyslexia* 32:33–60.

Markwardt, F. 1989. *Peabody Individual Achievement Test-Revised.* Circle Pines, MN: American Guidance Service.

Myklebust, H., and Boshes, B. 1969. *Minimal Brain Damage in Children.* Washington, DC: Department of Health, Education and Welfare, U.S.P.H.S.

Newcomer, P., and Hammill, D. 1982. *The Test of Language Development: Primary.* Austin, TX: PRO-ED.

Nurss, J. R., and McGauvran, M. E. 1986. *Metropolitan Readiness Test.* San Antonio, TX: Psychological Corporation.

Olson, R., Forsberg, H., Wise, B., and Rack, J. 1994. Measurement of word recognition, orthographic, and phonological skills. In *Frames of Reference for the Assessment of Learning Disabilities,* ed. G. R. Lyon, Baltimore: Brookes.

Richardson, E. 1985. *Decoding Skills Test.* Parkton, MD: York Press.

Rourke, B. 1989. *Nonverbal Learning Disabilities.* New York: Guilford.

Rutter, M. 1978. Dyslexia. In *Dyslexia: An Appraisal of Current Knowledge,* eds. A. Benton and D. Pearl. New York: Oxford University Press.

Shankweiler, D., and Liberman, I. 1972. Misreading: A search for causes. In *Language by Ear and by Eye,* eds. J. Kavanagh and L. Mattingly. Cambridge, MA: M.I.T. Press.

Siegel, L., and Ryan, E. 1984. Reading as a language disorder. *Remedial and special Education* 5(3):28–33.

Smith, S. 1994. *Different is Not Bad, Different is the World.* Longmont, CO: Sopris West.

Torgesen, J. K., and Bryant, B. R. 1994. *Test of Phonological Awareness.* Austin, TX: PRO-ED.

Vogel, S. 1975. *An Investigation of Syntactic Abilities in Normal and Dyslexic Children.* Baltimore, MD: University Park Press.

Wechsler, D. 1989. *Manual for the Wechsler Preschool and Primary Scale of Intelligence-Revised.* San Antonio: Psychological Corporation.

Wechsler, D. 1981. *Wechsler Adult Intelligence Scale-Revised.* San Antonio, TX: The Psychological Corporation.

Wechsler D. 1991. *Wechsler Intelligence Scale for Children-III.* New York: Psychological Corporation.

Wiederholt, J. L., and Bryant, B. R. 1992. *Gray Oral Reading Test* 3rd. ed. Austin, TX: PRO-ED.

Wiig, E. H., and Secord, W. 1989. *Test of Language Competence, Expanded Edition.* San Antonio, TX: Psychological Corporation.

Wilkinson, G. S. 1993. *Wide Range Achievement Test-3.* Wilmington, DE: Jastak Associates.

Wolf, M. 1984. Naming, reading and the dyslexias. A longitudinal overview. *Annals of Dyslexia* 34:87–115.

Woodcock, R. W., and Johnson, M. B. 1989. *Woodcock-Johnson Psychoeducational Battery-Revised.* Chicago, IL: Riverside Publishing.

Chapter • **8**

Dyslexia *Over- and* Under-*Diagnosis, Over- and* Under-*Sophistication*

Ruth Nass

Developmental dyslexia, an unexpected difficulty in learning to read (Symmes and Rapaport 1972), may be defined by both exclusionary and inclusionary criteria (Rudel 1980, 1985; Denckla 1993). The reading disabled subgroups uncovered by "violations" of some of the major traditional exclusionary criteria are examined here for the purpose of better understanding the neurobiology of dyslexia. With a similar goal, some less traditional potential inclusionary criteria are investigated.

TRADITIONAL EXCLUSIONARY CRITERIA

1. Based on strict definition, the dyslexic child may have *no major neurological abnormalities.* However, children with both congenital and acquired focal brain lesions do have reading problems. The frequency and location of the causative lesions provide information about the neuroanatomy of reading and the degree to which there is plasticity for recovery and reorganization in this domain. Children with acquired aphasia due to left hemisphere lesions generally recover conversational speech, but reading and spelling often remain difficult (Woods and Carey 1979; Levine, Hier, and Calvano 1981). Reading

deficits have also been reported with acquired right hemisphere lesions in childhood (Ferro et al. 1982; Martins, Ferro, and Trindade 1987). Children with pre-language acquisition cerebral lesions of either hemisphere will likely, but not necessarily, have reading and/or spelling difficulties (Daigneault, Braun, and Watters 1995; Nass and Stiles 1996). Those with *left subcortical* pathology may be at a particularly high risk (Aram, Gillespie, and Yamashita 1990). Ogden (1996), examining four adults with hemispherectomies after early unilateral brain damage, found that both left and right hemispherectomy patients could read regular and irregular learned words, but neither could spell nonwords. Unlike the right hemispherectomy patients, the left hemispherectomy patients were unable to read nonwords and to spell real words. The author thus suggests that aspects of phonology are the innate property of the left hemisphere. Innate specialization (Nass, Koch, and Peterson 1989), crowding (Levin and Scheller 1996), and computational biases (Bates, Thal, and Aram 1994), as well as the dynamics of reading acquisition itself (developmental changes in the linguistic/neuroanatomic correlates of reading achievement; Badian 1995; Fletcher 1981; Waterman and Lewandowski 1993; Frith 1986) may all play a role in bi-hemispheric lesion effects on reading. Reading qua multi-modal higher level skill may not be as amenable to the plasticity usually afforded to the immature nervous system.

The patterns of reading difficulties (words vs. non words; regular vs. irregular words) and types of errors (semantic, visual) in adults with acquired left hemisphere lesions (as they reflect the two major interacting routes to reading — visual and phonic) may have developmental equivalents (Malatesha and Aaron 1982; Malatesha and Whitaker 1984; Newcombe and Marshall 1984; Patterson, Marshall, and Coltheart 1985; Seymour 1992a, 1992b). Dyslexia can thereby be analyzed in terms of types of reading processing impairments.

There appear to be at least two ways to recognize a word: phonetically, letter by letter; or visually, by sight as a whole. Some children have trouble with the visual route to reading, with sight reading, and have been called "surface" or "dyseidetic" (Boder 1973) (unable to image the word) dyslexics. They cannot read irregular words that are not spelled the way they sound. Other children have trouble with the phonetic route to reading, sounding out, and have been termed "phonologic" or "dysphonetic" (Boder 1973) dyslexics. They cannot sound out unfamiliar words and cannot read phonetically regular non-words. In deep dyslexia both routes to reading are dysfunctional. When a word is read, the most common error is a semantic approximation of the test word suggesting some access into the lexicon, but with both input and output errors. Dyslexia may occur when a child fails to pass through any one of the stages of normal reading acquisition. The resultant subtypes (surface, phonological) provide information about the dynamics of the reading process per se (Roeltgen and Blaskey 1992; Frith 1986).

Generally, children with neurological impairment are excluded from studies of dyslexia. However, in comparing the reading of neurologically impaired (hydrocephalus, muscular dystrophy, mentally retarded) and non-neurologically impaired disabled readers, Mattis, French and Rapin (1975) found similar reading disability subtypes in each group (language disorder, visuo-perceptual disorder). These disability subtypes were not seen in the neurologically impaired readers. By contrast, Dorman (1987) found visuo-perceptual deficits, as well as Boder's (1973) subtype reading errors (dyseidetic-dysphonetic) in neurologically impaired students regardless of reading status (disabled or

Table I. Acquired and Developmental Dyslexias: Patterns of Deficits

	DEEP	PHONOLOGICAL	SURFACE
	imperfect direct lexical route	imperfect direct lexical route	imperfect indirect route
phonological system		↓↓↓↓ phonological assembly, parsed chunks too large	xs letter by letter parsed chunks too small
lexical system	↓	lexicalization of errors	↓
letter reading		↓ holistic approach	↓ e.g. reading disease as decrease
word vs. nonword	no nonwords read	nonwords much worse than words	regular words about = nonwords; nonwords > > irregular words
affect orthographic regularity	none	none	significant
homophone confusion	none	variable	marked
functor words	poor	variable	good
affect word length	none	variable	some effect
affect frequency	marked	variable–marked	slight
affect imageability	marked	variable	slight
lexican decision	good	variable	poor

surface = dyseidetic

↓ = decrease

xs = excess

Table II.   Error types in Acquired Dylsexias

	DEEP	PHONOLOGICAL	SURFACE
semantic rhyme → rhythm	++++	++	0
derivational variety → vary		++	
phonetic ought → out		+	
morphologic running → run	++	++	+
visual, B/P, M/N broad → board	+	+	+
visual/semantic acorn → wheat earl → deaf	+++	+	0
ortho-phonologic bike → bik, broad→ broke, break, braid	0	+/–	+++
phonemic regularization heir → hair			++

+ = frequency of error

+/– = sometimes

able). Thus, the issue of whether the associated cognitive deficits (language, visual spatial processing) are a general effect of neurologic impairment or a specific cause of the reading problem remains unresolved.

Although gross neurologic abnormalities are not present, the traditional dyslexic child may, and often does, have "soft signs" (Touwen and Prechtl 1970; Denckla 1977). Developmental soft signs are findings that would be normal if the child were younger (mirror movements, overflow). In Denckla's series, 38 of 52 children with pure dyslexia had such signs. Classic "pastel" soft signs are traditional neurologic signs found in a mild form (minimally asymmetric deep tendon reflexes). In Denckla's series, 11 of 52 had pastel signs. Both right and left hemisyndromes were demonstrated, although the side of the hemisyndrome did not correlate with the neuropsychological profile (language disorder vs. visuo-perceptual disorder). Only three of 52 children with pure dyslexia had no soft signs.

While language development and motor proficiency appear interrelated (Rudel 1985), fine motor disability in kindergarten, for example, does not predict dyslexia in second grade (Fletcher and Satz 1980) (table III). Notably, there is only minimal correlation between motor coordination on neurologic exams and athletic ability in the real world (Denckla 1985). The presence of co-morbid ADHD may have a significant effect on the number and types of soft signs on exam (Rudel 1985; Denckla 1985) (table IV). Reading disability with motor problems may be a specific inherited subtype of dyslexia (Rogehr and Kaplan 1988). Most investigators report a marked decline in the number of soft signs after puberty, but increasing the demands of the motor task brings out persisting difficulties in older dyslexics (Rousselle and Wolff 1991). Soft signs do not distinguish between an underlying left hemisphere deficit (apraxia) or reduced efficiency of interhemispheric transfer of information in dyslexia.

Not all children with dyslexia have soft signs. The manner and age at which neuropsychological signs are assessed may affect performance dramatically. In one large homogeneous sample, elementary school reading underachievers evidenced only a single soft sign. Although some dyslexics are poor copiers of designs, they may be very good judges of the accuracy of the copies (Benton and Pearl 1978). Many dyslexics miss the easy designs where precision counts, but get the harder ones where the concept counts (Denckla 1985). Perceptual motor deficits, like neurological soft signs, diminish in adolescents on some tasks (Beery's Visuo-Motor Integration Test, Semmes Map Walking, Rey Complex Figure [Denckla, Rudel, and Broman 1980; Denckla 1995]), perhaps reflecting right hemisphere

Table III.   Kindergarten Neurologic Examination

Task	Predict Second Grade Reading
Finger localization	yes
Alphabet recitation	yes
Recognition discrimination	yes
Verbal cognitive status	no
Fine motor status	no

Table IV.   Motor Skills: Dyslexics Vs. ADD (Denkla 1985)

	Dyslexics (pure)	ADD
Excess Overflow	no	yes
Slow FT, FS	only at 8 yrs	yes
Slow Feet	only at 7 and 8 yrs	yes, yes
Slow Learn, Effortful	yes	
Large R-L Differences	yes	
Slow Left Side	yes	
Left Pantomime Problems	yes	
Asymmetric Left→Right Mirroring	yes	

FT = finger tapping
FS = finger sequencing

"hypertrophy." The great art of Leonardo DiVinci or the music of John Lennon may exemplify this.

2) The major sensory functions must be normal; the traditional dyslexic child *cannot be blind or deaf*. Notably, deaf children have more difficulty learning to read than blind children, presumably because the former lack the necessary language background /phonological awareness. Despite the theoretical appeal of the recent proposal that visual processing by a "slow" lateral geniculate magnocellular system (important for monitoring motion, stereopsis, spatial localization, depth and figure/ground perception) does not appropriately modify the information received from the parvocellular system (crucial for color perception, object recognition, and high resolution form perception), the evoked potential responses initially reported in support of this hypothesis have not been replicated (Livingstone et al. 1991; Victor et al. 1993). Recent studies using magneto-encephalography (MEEG) (Salmelin et al. 1996) and positron emission tomography (PET) scanning (Eden et al. 1996) have, however, provided some support for this theory. The proposed remediations (reduce contrast, use diffuse color lights/ lenses), which variably inhibit magno and parvocellular systems, do not have proven efficacy (Menacker et al. 1993).

3) *Normal intelligence* is a requirement for a traditional diagnosis. (See Siegel 1989, 1992 for further discussion as to whether an IQ discrepancy is relevant to the inclusionary diagnosis of dyslexia.) Verbal intelligence is often considered a potentially biased measure since many children with dyslexia have a history of language delay. Yet, the child with persisting language problems (and impaired Verbal IQ) probably should not be diagnosed as dyslexic in the strict sense. Rather, the reading difficulty here is an extension of the language problem, as opposed to a problem in and of itself. This caveat would apply to Tallal's population with processing-rate-based developmental language disorders and concurrent dyslexia. Indeed, Tallal, Miller and Fitch (1993), comparing dyslexics with and without persisting oral language impairments, found that those with oral language impairments had deficits in nonsense word reading and non-verbal temporal processing, while those without oral language impairments had neither phonological decoding deficits nor temporal processing deficits in any sensory modality.

Also of note relative to the intelligence and reading debate, Mattis et al. (1977) found both readers and non-readers in their mentally retarded control group.

4) The dyslexic child must have been in a *social and educational environment conducive to learning to read*. Studies of inner-city elementary school children demonstrate that enrichment programs can help

some non-readers become readers. For example, inner-city elementary school non-reading students were taught and learned a set of Chinese characters over a short period of time (Rozin, Poritsky, and Sotsky 1980). Whether the lack of phonics in this particular reading task or whether the extra attention contributed to the students' success is not determinable. Reading to children during elementary school has been documented to accelerate reading acquisition.

Instructional variables, even in the ordinary early elementary school classroom, are an important factor differentiating reading difficulties from dyslexia (Vellutino in press). If different amounts of time are spent on language arts, and decoding and reading for meaning in different classrooms in the same school, how can one tell educational effects from biology? Even teaching approaches that explicitly encourage phonics vary as to the particular unit of sound on which reading instruction is based (Snowling 1996).

NON-TRADITIONAL INCLUSIONARY CRITERIA

With respect to possible *inclusionary criteria, reading two grades behind* actual or expected grade level is generally required for a diagnosis of dyslexia by educational authorities (Badian 1996). Investigation of some less traditional criteria yield some interesting information about what dyslexia actually is.

1. The "two grades behind" criterion does not take into account that, because of the complex dynamics of reading acquisition, *different types of reading tests* yield different reading levels and may be more or less reliable measures and predictors of reading ability at different ages or grade levels. For example, Rudel (1980) found that some children had trouble on the Gray Oral Reading Test, which is timed and requires comprehension of what is read, but did not have trouble on the Wide Range Achievement Test, a single word reading test that only requires phonetic decoding (particularly if decoding was the emphasis of tutoring) (Rudel 1980). Other children have significant difficulties with phonologic awareness (Stanovitch and Siegel 1994) and segmentation, leading, for example, to low Word Attack scores. However, if children are bright and get clues from context, their silent reading comprehension may be at grade or above. Badian (1995) found that different cognitive/ reading/ spelling skills in preschool and grades one and three predicted sixth grade reading ability (table V).

2. The *age of the child* affects the inclusionary criteria. Because we do not expect children to read until first grade, the strict definition makes a diagnosis of dyslexia impossible before the third grade. Yet a

Table V.

Predictors of Grade 6 Reading Differ by Age:
Preschool predictors:
Letter naming; visual matching; visual motor
Grade 1 predictors
Test of Auditory Analysis Skills (syllables; phonemes)
Spelling hard: elephant, beauty, potato, holiday, listen
Pseudo-spelling easy:ot, sug, hib, eft, lan, pund, timp, frot, mest, plag
Grade 3 predictors
Pseudo-spelling easy and hard: feem, shipe, blowk
Garl, scrage, sproke, graif, cherg, thraup, ploog
Badian 1995

history of language delay is often predictive of dyslexia (Rapin 1982; Mann 1992) and strict adherence to definition should not preempt consideration of early intervention (Badian 1988; Lundberg 1996). In addition, a two-year discrepancy reflects a greater disability for the younger than for the older child.

3. Several *cognitive models* of developmental dyslexia including: clustering (Rourke and Orr 1977), clinical observation of neuropsychological strength/weakness profiles (Mattis et al. 1977; Denckla 1977), and linguistic analysis (Boder 1973; Roeltgen 1992; and Seymour 1992 a and b) have been proposed. Considering them in the inclusionary criteria for the diagnosis of dyslexia would certainly enhance our understanding of the neural modules involved in the reading process. For example, Hynd and Semrud-Clikeman (1989), Hynd (1995), and Semrud-Clikeman et al. (1991) found that different reading deficits were associated with different structural abnormalities of the brain (table VI). Hier and colleagues (1978) found that the lowest verbal and reading scores were seen in those dyslexics with atypical planum temporale asymmetries.

4. *Spelling* disability may be a mild form of reading disability (Share et al. 1987; Finucci et al. 1982) or a residual of prior dyslexia in adulthood (Finucci et al. 1984). Whether the two are dissociable (sound-to-spell different from spell-to-sound) or based on the same un-

Table VI. Dyslexic (D) Vs. ADD Vs. Controls (Hynd and Semrud-Clikeman 1989)

↓R frontal width ↓passage comprehension (D only)
Atypical anterior asymmetry ↓word attack (D only)
Atypical planum ↓verbal comprehension (All Groups)
Atypical callosum (ADD, D)

↓ = decreased

derlying phonological ability is debated (Frith 1980; Roeltgen 1992). Frith proposes that early logographic reading revolves around a sight word vocabulary dependent on salient graphic features (major consonants); context; pragmatics; and guessing, largely ignoring letter order. This is followed by alphabetic reading using individual grapheme/phoneme correspondences—letter-by-letter reading. Here phonemic segmentation, letter order, and phonology are important, but there is little semantics. Mature reading is orthographic—instant analysis of words by orthographic units without phonologic conversion, which coincides with morpheme or other sublexical representations. Unexpected poor spelling in adolescence may reflect good alphabetic/phonologic ability, but impaired orthographic processing. Skills are good enough for reading, but not sufficient for spelling

Phonological awareness is probably even more important for spelling than reading. Children spell words they cannot read until the age of 10. Early spelling helps early reading; later reading helps the development of visual memory for words, which then results in improved spelling (table VII). Presence of spelling difficulties (and subtle phonological problems) in adults with a history of developmental dyslexia and in families with genetically based reading disabilities (Pennington 1986) support the relevance of spelling to the definition of dyslexia per se.

In summation, although our understandings of the biological basis of dyslexia is rapidly evolving (Rumsey et al. 1992, 1994a, 1994b; Hynd 1995), the formal definition of dyslexia requires continuing scrutiny.

Table VII   Frith's Model of Reading and Spelling Acquisition

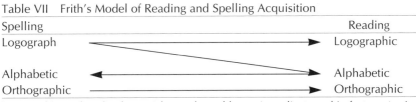

Spelling	Reading
Logograph	Logographic
Alphabetic	Alphabetic
Orthographic	Orthographic

Logographic readers develop a sight word vocablary using salient graphic features (major consonants), context, pragmatics, and guessing. They largely ignore letter order.

Alphabetic readers use individual graphemes and phonemes and their correspondences. They read letter-by-letter, use phonemic segmentation, letter order, and phonology. Semantics plays little role in reading.

Orthographic readers instantly analyze words by orthographic units (letter combinations) without phonologic conversion.

REFERENCES

Aram, D., Gillespie, L., and Yamashita, T. 1990. Reading among children with left and right brain lesions. *Developmental Neuropsychology* 6:301–17.

Badian, N. 1995. Predicting reading ability over the long term. *Annals of Dyslexia* 45:79–98.

Badian, N. 1996. Dyslexia: A validation of the concept at two grade levels. *Journal of Learning Disabilities* 29:102–12.

Badian, N. 1988. Predicting dyslexia in the preschool population. In *Preschool Prevention of Reading Failure*, eds. R. L. Masland, and M. W. Masland. Parkton, MD: York Press.

Bates, E., Thal, D., Aram, D., Fenson, J., Trauner, D., Eisele, J., and Nass, R. 1994. From first words to grammar after early focal lesions. *Developmental Psychology*, 10:222–44.

Benton, A., and Pearl, D. (eds.) 1978. *Dyslexia: An Appraisal of Current Knowledge*. New York: Oxford Press.

Boder, E. 1973. Developmental dyslexia: A diagnostic approach based on three atypical reading-spelling patterns. *Developmental Medicine Child Neurology* 15:663–87.

Daigneault, S., Braun, C., and Watters, G. 1995. Alexia following a perinatal left temporal lesion: Evidence of a module for the acquisition of reading. *Journal of the International Neuropsychology Society* 23:15.

Denckla, M. 1985. Motor coordination in dyslexic children. In *Dyslexia*, eds. F. Duffy and N. Geschwind. Boston: Little, Brown.

Denckla, M.B., Rudel, R., and Broman, M. 1980. The development of a spatial orientation skill in normal, learning-disabled, and neurologically impaired children. In *Biological Studies of Mental Processes*, ed. D. Caplan. Cambridge, MA: MIT Press.

Denckla, M.B. 1977. Dyslexia. In *Topics in Child Neurology*, eds. M. Blaw, I. Rapin, and M. Kinsbourne. New York: Spectrum Press.

Denckla, M.B. 1993. A neurologist's overview of developmental dyslexia. In *Temporal Information Processing in the Nervous System*, eds. P. Tallal, A. M. Galaburda, R. R. Llinás, and C. von Euler. New York: New York Academy of Sciences.

Dorman, C. 1987. Reading disability subtypes in neurologically impaired children. *Annals of Dyslexia* 37:166–88.

Eden, G., VanMeter, J., Rumsey, J., Maisog, J., Woods, R., and Zeffiro, T. 1996. Abnormal processing of visual motion in dyslexia revealed by functional brain imaging. *Nature* 382:66–69.

Ferro, J., Martins, I., Pinto, F., and Castro-Caldas, A. 1982. Aphasia following right striato-insular infarction in a left handed child. *Developmental Medicine Child Neurology* 24:173–82.

Finucci, J., Whitehouse, C., Isaacs, S., and Childs, B. 1984. Derivation and validation of a quantitative definition of specific reading disability for adults. *Developmental Medicine Child Neurology* 26:143–53.

Finucci, J., Isaacs, S., Whitehouse, C., and Childs, B. 1982. Empirical validation of reading and spelling quotients. *Developmental Medicine Child Neurology* 24:733–44.

Fletcher, J. 1981. Linguistic factors in reading acquisition: Evidence for developmental change. *Neuropsychological and Cognitive Processes in Reading.* New York: Academic Press.

Fletcher, J., and Satz, P. 1980. Developmental changes in the linguistic performance correlates of reading achievement. *Journal of Clinical Psychology* 2:23–37.

Frith, U. 1986. A developmental framework for developmental dyslexia. *Annals of Dyslexia* 36:69–81.

Frith, U. (ed.) 1980. *Cognitive Processes in Spelling.* London: Academic Press.

Hier, D. B., LeMay, M., Rosenberger, P. B., and Perlo, V. P. 1978. Developmental dyslexia: Evidence for a subgroup with reversed cerebral asymmetry. *Archives of Neurology* 35:90–92.

Hynd, G., and Semrud-Clikeman, M. 1989. Dyslexia and brain morphology. *Psychological Bulletin* 106:447–82.

Hynd, G. 1995. Dyslexia and corpus callosum morphology. *Archives of Neurology* 92:32–38.

Johannes, S., Kussmaul, C., Munte, T., and Mangun, G. 1996. Developmental dyslexia: Passive visual stimulation provides no evidence for a magnocellular processing deficit. *Neuropsychologia* 34:1123–27.

Levin, H., and Scheller, J. 1996. Dyscalculia and dyslexia after right hemisphere injury. *Archives of Neurology* 53:88–96.

Levine, D. N., Hier, D. B., and Calvano, R. 1981. Acquired learning disability for reading after left temporal lobe damage in childhood. *Neurology* 31:257–64.

Livingstone, M., Rosen, G., Drislane, F. I., and Galaburda, A. 1991. Physiological and anatomical evidence for a magnocellular defect in developmental dyslexia. *Proceedings of the National Academy of Science* 88:7943–47.

Lundberg, I. 1996. Reading difficulties can be predicted and prevented. In *Reading Development and Dyslexia,* eds. C. Hume and M. Snowling. London: Whurr.

Malatesha, R., and Aaron, P. (eds.) 1982. *Reading Disorders.* New York: Academic Press.

Malatesha, R., and Whitaker, H. (eds.) 1984. *Dyslexia: A Global Issue.* The Hague: Martinus Nijhoff Publishers.

Mann, V. 1992. Language problems: A key to early reading problems. In *Learning About Learning Disabilities,* ed. B. Wong. San Diego: Academic Press.

Martins, I., Ferro, J., and Trindade, A. 1987. Acquired crossed aphasia in a child. *Developmental Medicine Child Neurology* 29:96–100.

Mattis, S., French, J., and Rapin, I. 1975. Dyslexia in children and young adults. Three independent neuropsychological syndromes. *Developmental Medicine Child Neurology* 17:150–63.

Menacker, S., Breton, M., Radcliffe, J., and Gole, G. 1993. Do tinted lens improve the reading performance of dyslexic children? *Archives Ophthalmology* 111:213–18.

Nass, R., Peterson, H., and Koch, D. 1989. Differential effects of early left versus right brain injury on intelligence. *Brain and Cognition* 9:258–66.

Nass, R., and Stiles, J. 1996. Cognitive complications of the perinatum: Congenital focal lesions. In *Pediatric Behavioral Neurology,* ed. Y. Frank. Boca Raton, FL: CRC Press.

Newcombe, F., and Marshall, J. 1984. Varieties of acquired dyslexia: A linguistic approach. *Seminars Neurology* 4:181–91.

Ogden J. 1996. Phonological dyslexia and phonological dysgraphia following left and right hemispherectomy. *Neuropsychologia* 34:905–18.

Patterson, K., Marshall, J., and Coltheart, M. 1985. *Surface Dyslexia*. Hillsdale, NJ: Lawrence Erlbaum Associates.

Pennington, B. 1986. Spelling errors in adults with a form of familial dyslexia. *Child Development* 57:1001–13.

Rapin, I. 1982. Developmental language disorders and brain dysfunction as precursors of reading disability. In *Topics in Child Neurology*, Vol. 2, eds. G. A. Wise, M. E. Blaw, and P. G. Procopis. New York: Spectrum Publications.

Roeltgen, D., and Blaskey, P. 1992. Processes, breakdowns, and remediation in developmental disorders of reading and spelling. In *Cognitive Neuropsychology in Clinical Practice*, ed. D. Margolin. New York: Oxford.

Roeltgen, D. 1992. Phonological error analysis, development and empirical evaluation. *Brain and Language* 22:807–20.

Rogehr, S., and Kaplan, B. 1988. Reading disability with motor problems may be an inherited subtype. *Pediatrics* 82:204–10.

Rourke, B., and Orr, R. 1977. Prediction of reading and spelling performance of normal and retarded readers: A four-year follow-up. *Journal of Abnormal Child Psychology* 5:9–15.

Rousselle, C., and Wolff, P. 1991. The dynamics of bimanual coordination in developmental dyslexia. *Neuropsychologia* 29:907–24.

Rozin, P., Poritsky, S., and Sotsky, R. 1987. American children with reading problems can easily learn to read English representation by Chinese characters. *Science* 272:1264–67.

Rudel, R. 1985. The definition of dyslexia: Language and motor deficits. In *Dyslexia*, eds. F. Duffy and N. Geschwind. Boston: Little Brown.

Rudel, R. 1980. Learning disability: Diagnosis by exclusion and discrepancy. *Journal of the American Academy of Child Psychiatry* 19:547–78.

Rumsey, J. M., Andreason, P., Zametkin, A. J., Hamburger, S. D., Aquino, T., King, A. C., Pikus, A., Rapaport, J., and Cohen, R. M. 1994a. Right fronto-temporal activation by tonal memory in dyslexia. A ^{15}O PET study. *Biological Psychiatry* 36:171–80.

Rumsey, J. M., Andreason, P., Zametkin, A. J., Hamburger, S. D., Aquino, T., King, A. C., Pikus, A., Rapaport, J., and Cohen, R. M. 1994b. Normal activation of frontotemporal language cortex in dyslexia: A ^{15}O PET study. *Archives of Neurology* 51:27–38.

Rumsey, J., Andreason, P., Zametkin, A. J., Hamburger, S. D., Aquino, T., King, A. C., Pikus, A., Rapaport, J., and Cohen, R. M. 1992. Failure to activate left temporoparietal cortex in dyslexia : A ^{15}O PET study. *Archives of Neurology* 49:527–34.

Salmelin, R., Service, E., Kiesila, P., Uutela, K., and Salonen, O. 1996. Impaired visual word processing in dyslexia revealed by MEEG. *Annals of Neurology* 40:157–62.

Semrud-Clikeman, M., Hynd, G., Novey, E., and Eliopulos, D. 1991. Dyslexia and brain morphology. *Learning and Individual Differences* 3:225–42.

Seymour, P. 1992a. The assessment of reading disorders. In *A Handbook of Neuropsychological Assessment*, eds. J. Crawford, D. Parker, and W. McKinlay. Hillsdale, NJ: Lawrence Erlbaum Associates.

Seymour, P. 1992b. Developmental dyslexia: A cognitive experimental analysis. In *Cognitive Neuropsychology in Clinical Practice,* ed. D. I. Margolin. New York: Oxford.

Share, D., Silva, P., and Adler, C. 1987. Factors associated with reading-plus-spelling retardation and specific spelling retardation. *Developmental Medicine Child Neurology* 29:72–84.

Siegel, L. 1992. An evaluation of the discrepancy diagnosis of dyslexia. *Journal of Learning Disabilities* 25:618–37.

Siegel, L. 1989. IQ is irrelevant to the definition of learning disabilities. *Journal of Learning Disabilities* 22:469–77.

Snowling, M. 1996. Annotation: Contemporary approaches to the teaching of reading. *Journal of Child Psychology and Psychiatry* 37:139–48.

Stanovitch, K., and Siegel, L. 1994. The phenotypic performance profile of reading disabled children. *Journal of Educational Psychology* 86:1–30.

Symmes, J., and Rapaport, J. 1972. Unexpected reading failure. *American Journal of Orthopsychiatry* 42:82–8.

Tallal, P., Miller, S., and Fitch, R. 1993. Neurobiological basis of speech. In *Temporal Information Processing in the Nervous System,* eds. P. Tallal, A. Galaburda, R. R. Llinás, and C. von Euler. New York: New York Academy of Sciences.

Touwen, B., and Prechtl, H. 1970. *Neurological Examination in Minimal Brain Dysfunction.* London: Spastics International.

Vellutino, F. In press. Cognitive profile of difficult to remediate and readily remediated poor readers: Early intervention as a vehicle for distinguishing between cognitive and experiential deficits as basic causes of reading disability. *Journal of Educational Psychology.*

Victor, J., Conte, M., Burton, L., and Nass, R. 1993. Lack of visual evoked response potential evidence for magnocellular dysfunction in dyslexia. *Visual Neuroscience* 10:939–46.

Waterman, B., and Lewandowski, L. 1993. Phonological and semantic processing in reading-disabled and non-disabled males at two age levels. *Journal of Experimental Child Psychology* 55:87–103.

Woods, T., and Carey, S. 1979. Language deficits after apparent clinical recovery from childhood aphasia. *Annals of Neurology* 6:405–9.

Section • IV

Management of Specific Reading Disability

Chapter • 9

Diagnosis and Remediation of Dyslexia

Robin P. Church,
Marjorie A. Fessler, and
Michael Bender

This chapter attempts to address the parameters involved in assessing this distinct learning disability while providing suggestions for appropriate classroom interventions.

Although a great amount of literature is currently available in the domain of assessment, we point out the necessity first to define the reason for evaluating a specific individual, and then to place the information from an assessment into context; that is, in terms of remediation or placement or as data for developing specific clinical evidence.

In reading this chapter, it quickly becomes clear that assessment is a multifaceted process which, in most instances, provides a framework for making future recommendations. Because not all tests are created equal, it is critical that tests and procedures be selected with the utmost care in terms of answering questions and making useful comparisons. Traditionally, medical, developmental, and educational histories form the base from which assessment begins. These domains are briefly explained and provide measurable pieces of information for identifying initial reading acquisition milestones.

The role of cognitive profiles is also examined in this chapter, especially since IQ-reading discrepancy continues to be used as a way of documenting dyslexia for placement purposes. Of equal importance is a discussion of phonological processing skills as a critical domain for investigation of individuals with suspected dyslexia. Tests that purport to assess rapid naming deficits, verbal short-term memory, phonological awareness, and sound blending are also discussed in the context of their uses in diagnosing dyslexia.

Although the determination of whether or not a student may be dyslexic is not always clear, what is clear is an immediate need for appropriate school placement and interventions. Like assessment, interventions can run the gamut, and the selection of one over another may often depend on a specific teacher's or team's advocacy. For the reader who may require some basic introductory information concerning how students acquire reading skills, three major conceptual models are presented: the top-down processing model, the bottom-up processing model, and the interactive model.

How does dyslexia appear to the classroom teacher? Is it in the context of a reading disorder or does it also include related problems in the areas of spelling, written expression, handwriting, reading rate, or phonological processing? It is also critical to point out that most classes have twenty-five or more students seeking a teacher's attention which leaves little time for special attention or help.

Intervention can take many forms, be it direct instruction, mastery learning, or multisensory learning. Regardless of the form, remediating dyslexia requires instruction in weaker areas while building on strengths. Information about instructional approaches and programs is provided in the chapter, including cooperative learning strategies which have added an additional instructional tool for reading disabled students who may be in inclusion or general education classes. The reader is urged to seek out contemporary software and resources found in libraries and over the Internet. In this way, the search for new assessment ideas and remedial techniques will parallel the expanding needs of students with dyslexia.

ASSESSMENT OF DYSLEXIA

At the outset, it is necessary to clarify whether the purpose of assessment is for research or practical purposes. Those involved in research of individuals with dyslexia require clear parameters for determining membership in a sample population. On the other hand, those concerned with appropriate placement and instructional programs for students with dyslexia must address more practical issues. A recent working definition of dyslexia, developed by The Orton Dyslexia Society Research Committee in April 1994, may provide guidance to researchers, clinicians, teachers, and parents in understanding the multiple factors that should be considered in its diagnosis.

> Dyslexia is one of several distinct learning disabilities. It is a specific language-based disorder of constitutional origin, characterized by difficulties in single word decoding, usually reflecting insufficient phonological processing. These difficulties in single word decoding are often unexpected in relation to age and other cognitive and academic abilities; they are not the result of generalized developmental disability or sensory impairment. Dyslexia is manifested by variable difficulty with different forms of language, often including, in addition to problems with reading, a conspicuous problem with acquiring proficiency in writing and spelling.

The first statement of this definition reflects accruing research and clinical evidence that individuals with dyslexia often display concurrent difficulties in other cognitive and academic areas, such as attention (Shankweiler et al. 1995); mathematics (Fletcher and Loveland 1986); and spelling and written expression (Lindamood 1994; Moats 1994). Other aspects of the definition denote the need to (a) explore medical, developmental, and educational histories through interview; (b) obtain cognitive profiles and compare reading achievement with a variety of cognitive measures; (c) assess performance between and within academic domains on standardized achievement tests; and (d) measure phonological processing skills. Use of curriculum-based and criterion-referenced instruments, observation, and clinical teaching to inventory reading skills and strategies is also critical in determining appropriate and effective prescriptive/remedial techniques.

Assessment provides a framework for testing hypotheses about the presence of dyslexia. Although professionals should attempt to gather information from a variety of sources using multiple methods, clearly they should be discriminating in their selection of assessment tools. Tests and procedures should be selected to (a) answer specific questions and (b) provide a baseline against which future growth can be measured (Clark and Uhry 1995).

Medical, Developmental, and Educational Histories

Much like physicians, who derive considerable information from interviewing their patients, those assessing dyslexia may use this technique to obtain information from parents, teachers, and students themselves.

Medical and Developmental Issues. Increasingly, researchers are finding that dyslexia "runs" in families, may be inherited , and could reflect autosomal dominant transmission (DeFries 1991; Olson 1989; Olson

1990; Pennington 1995). Parents often report to clinicians that multiple family members, including themselves, have poor reading skills and/or attentional problems. Parents with these disorders often recognize the importance of reading, but their own reading failures may deter them from reading to their children regularly or providing early phonological awareness activities that stimulate reading development.

The developmental history may also reveal factors that affect acquisition of reading skills. For example, children with delays in speech and language development may be at risk for later reading problems (Johnson and Croasmun 1991; Stark et al. 1984). Notable medical events, such as radiation or chemotherapy treatment for cancer, put children at increased risk for dyslexia and other learning disabilities (Brown and Modan-Swain 1993).

Educational History. Interviewers should obtain information about students' attendance records and the number of schools they have attended to rule out other possible causes of reading problems. Lack of instruction due to prolonged absences during critical periods in reading acquisition (Clark and Uhry 1995) or inconsistent reading instruction resulting from frequent changes in schools adversely affect student achievement.

Parent, teacher, and student interviews often yield important information about past and current academic progress, prior and current reading approaches, and reading techniques that have proved ineffective. Students with dyslexia typically have a history of poor academic achievement dating from their kindergarten years; for example, they may have trouble learning letter names and sounds (Fawcett and Nicolson 1994), reciting the alphabet or writing it, and acquiring a bank of basic sight words (Olson et al. 1989). Lacking in basic phonological awareness skills, they may not successfully demonstrate effective decoding strategies needed for reading fluency. Parents often report that their children read dysfluently and inconsistently, pausing each time they encounter words that seem unfamiliar, or failing to recognize words that they have successfully decoded earlier on the same page. In the classroom, use of intensive, individualized, and structured intervention strategies for teaching effective decoding skills, automatization of sight word recognition, and phonological skills training is often cited as the cornerstone of reading success (Adams 1990; Adams and Bruck 1995; Beck and Juel 1995). Parents and teachers often turn to private tutors, tutorial agencies, or packaged programs to supplement school-based instruction.

Compilation of an educational history, in combination with medical and developmental history, is helpful in generating hypothe-

ses about reading failure and facilitates the selection of appropriate assessment methods and instruments.

Cognitive Profiles

Despite the controversy that has raged in the research literature regarding the use of IQ-reading discrepancy to diagnose dyslexia
(Fletcher 1992; Fletcher et al. 1994; Olson et al. 1989; Siegel 1989;
Stanovich and Siegel 1994), it is still common practice nationwide to
document such discrepancies when decisions are made about eligibility for special education services in the public schools. Most school
districts use the Full Scale IQ or instruments such as the Wechsler
Intelligence Scale for Children-Third Edition (Wechsler 1991), unless
the Verbal and Performance Scale IQ scores are significantly discrepant. In the event of such a discrepancy, typically the higher score
is used as the most representative measure of cognition.

Clark and Uhry (1995) advocate use of the Verbal Scale IQ, indicating that an IQ score of 85 or above, in contrast to discrepant word
reading and other verbal abilities, is a key element in documenting
"evidence of specific reading-related weakness in the presence of statistically stronger oral comprehension" (p. 49). They state that a finding of low reading and high Verbal Scale IQ indicates a bright child
with dyslexia. In contrast, low reading and Verbal Scale IQ scores, in
combination with a high Performance Scale IQ score, indicates a
bright child with a language disorder. Concurrent low scores on measures of reading and Full Scale IQ suggest overall low reading and
academic performance—the "garden variety" poor reader described
by Stanovich (1991).

As proposed by Siegel (1989), there is evidence that the relationship between achievement and IQ is likely bi-directional (Shaywitz et
al. 1992). Findings from clinical practice suggest that IQ scores can decline over time when children do not read. Poor readers do not acquire
the vocabulary and knowledge base needed to respond successfully to
more difficult questions on IQ tests. This phenomenon, concomitant
drops in performance on both reading and IQ measures, often results
in children, previously diagnosed as dyslexic, becoming ineligible for
special education services as they get older.

Given the problem inherent in the IQ-reading discrepancy
model, it is necessary for clinicians and school-based professionals to
use multiple measures to diagnose dyslexia. Building a cognitive profile may include results of IQ assessment, but should also address cognitive processing and problem-solving skills (e.g., immediate and
working memory, vocabulary, verbal and nonverbal reasoning, visual

processing, auditory processing, and ability to benefit from instruction). Tests that comprehensively measure these areas include the Woodcock-Johnson Psycho-Educational Battery-Revised (Woodcock and Johnson 1990), the Swanson Cognitive Processing Test (Swanson 1996), and the Detroit Tests of Learning Aptitude-3 (Hammill 1991).

Assessment of Performance Between and Within Academic Domains

Practitioners and researchers often seek evidence of discrepancies between and within content domains to support the hypothesis of dyslexia. A widely used method, promulgated by Stanovich (1991) to avoid the use of IQ tests, is the comparison of student performance on tests of listening comprehension and reading comprehension. In using standardized measures, it is important to select the listening and reading comprehension subtests from the same battery (e.g., the Wechsler Individual Achievement Test, Wechsler 1992) to assure that they have been normed on the same sample. Such measures routinely reflect performance over a number of passages in each area. While informal comparisons of reading and listening comprehension have commonly been used by reading clinicians and teachers, these measures typically consist of one or two passages in each area. These passages are more susceptible to students' reliance on idiosyncratic background knowledge rather than on text knowledge to answer questions correctly (Clark and Uhry 1995). Gough (Gough and Tunmer 1986), in addressing the comparison of listening and reading comprehension, suggests that students who understand spoken text better than text that they must read, have deficits in word reading.

A more direct emphasis on single word reading has been espoused by multiple researchers (Adams 1990; Adams and Bruck 1995; Beck and Juel 1995; Olson et al. 1994; Shankweiler and Liberman 1989; Stanovich 1990; Stanovich and Siegel 1994) in diagnosing dyslexia. Their findings suggest that rapid and accurate word recognition is a prerequisite to understanding what is read. Essentially, "when word recognition processes demand too much cognitive capacity, few cognitive resources are left to allocate to higher-level processes of text integration and comprehension" (Lyon 1995, pp. 14–15). Olson and colleagues (1994) advocate use of computer-generated lists of words so that both accuracy and speed of response can be measured. They issue a cautionary note about the use of commercial tests, suggesting that the word lists on them may not be sufficiently long to avoid the influence of students' idiosyncratic knowledge.

Clark and Uhry (1995) suggest comparison of decoding and comprehension as an alternative method of pinpointing word reading problems. Their findings indicate that older, remediated students with dyslexia often can understand text at levels commensurate with their age, IQ, and listening ability, but continue to decode "somewhat inaccurately and extremely slowly" (p. 50). A discrepancy between decoding and comprehension, in such cases, supports the presence of a decoding disorder. Dr. Martha Bridge Denckla, in her discussions of clinical cases, has referred to these students as "deep dyslexics" in that they can correctly answer questions about passages despite misreading more than 50% of the words (personal communication, March 15, 1995).

Students with dyslexia often are more proficient at reading real words than nonsense words based on phonetically and orthographically regular patterns (Rack, Snowling, and Olson 1992). In making such comparisons, it is important to use tests normed on the same population (e.g., the Word Attack and Letter-Word Identification subtest of the Woodcock-Johnson Psycho-Educational Battery-Revised: Tests of Achievement). A mechanism for exploring this discrepancy is found on the Decoding Skills Test (Richardson and DiBennedetto 1985).

Since young students with dyslexia tend to be poor spellers who remain so even after their decoding of real words improves, some researchers have proposed use of spelling measures with high reliability and broad samplings of orthographic and morphologic patterns (Moats 1994). A different method, advocated by Lindamood, suggests use of the Lindamood Auditory Conceptualization Test (Lindamood and Lindamood 1979) to examine spelling without using letters at all. In clinical and school settings, the WIAT spelling subtest (Wechsler 1992) has been suggested because of its balance of word types, its reliability, and its comparisons of spelling performance with word reading, reading comprehension, and listening comprehension on the same measure (Clark and Uhry 1995).

Finally, discrepancies between achievement in reading and math are often used to support the hypothesis of a specific, as compared to general, learning disorder. Students with dyslexia often perform well on measures of math, especially math reasoning, but do poorly in reading. Those with poor automatic retrieval skills may have trouble with both decoding and recall of basic math facts, leading to limited skill development in word recognition and calculation. If practitioners wish to use standardized batteries of tests for comparisons, they are urged to select tests/subtests with high reliability (preferably .90 or higher) that are normed on the same sample (Berk 1982; Berk 1984; Hill 1981).

It is possible to profile reading and spelling scores that reflect the characteristics of older students who have received remediation, according to a model developed by Clark and Uhry (1995). Their scores indicate that listening comprehension > reading comprehension > decoding words in text > decoding words in isolation > spelling/nonsense word reading.

Assessment of Phonological Processing Skills

Increasingly, current models of reading disability implicate phonological processing as the critical domain of impairment in students with dyslexia (Jorm 1983; Stanovich 1988). Typically, three components of phonological processing are mentioned: rapid automatized or serial naming, verbal short-term memory, and phonological awareness. The literature suggests that all three are related to dyslexia, and that each can be present in the absence of the other two (Clark and Uhry 1995).

Rapid Automatized (Serial) Naming. The Rapid Automatized Naming Test (RAN), developed by Denckla and Rudel (1974), is used to assess rapid serial naming skills. On this measure, students are asked to name colors, single-digit numerals, depicted objects, and lower case alphabet letters. For each subtest, the five stimuli are presented in random order on 50-item matrices. Students are encouraged to name each set of stimuli as rapidly as possible, and are timed as they execute each task. Norms for each subtest permit clinicians to compare individual students' retrieval of labels with that of age peers. Evidence of slow retrieval alone, does not construe dyslexia, but rather is used as part of a student profile of skills. In clinical settings, findings suggest that performances of one to two standard deviations below peers on more than one RAN subtest is common in students with severe and persistent difficulty acquiring speed in decoding (Clark and Uhry 1995). Recent research has also indicated that rapid naming deficits often persist into adulthood in individuals diagnosed with dyslexia (Wood et al.1991).

Verbal Short-Term Memory. There are several alternatives to measuring verbal short-term memory, but little agreement about the optimal method. Some use the Digit Span subtest from the WISC-III, which requires the student to repeat digits in forward and reverse order. This method allows the professional to compare performance on Digit Span with other subtests of the Verbal Scale of the WISC-III. Another alternative is to use subtests from the Woodcock-Johnson Psycho-Educational Battery-Revised: Tests of Cognitive Ability so that memory for rote material (e.g., digits reversed or lists of unrelated words) can be compared to memory for meaningful material (e.g., words in sentence form). Standard scores from the Digits Reversed and/or Memory for Words subtests may be compared to findings from the Memory for Sentences subtest. As with the RAN results, difficulties with verbal short-term memory do not independently suggest dyslexia, but may be included in a profile of skills to clarify areas of strength and weakness.

Phonological Awareness. The relationship between phonological awareness and early reading has been long standing, dating to the 1970s (Adams 1990). Phonological awareness is best defined as "metacognitive understanding that spoken language is made up of a series of sounds and that these sounds occupy a particular sequential order" (Clark and Uhry 1995, p. 30).

Several measures have been developed to assess phonological awareness. One of the most recent is the Test of Phonological Awareness (Torgesen and Bryant 1994). This is a screening test designed for students in grades K-2, that requires matching pictures to words by initial or final sound. Sawyer's Test of Awareness of Language Segments (1987) has students use colored blocks to segment oral language, moving from segmentation of words in sentences, to syllables in words, to phonemes in single syllables (Clark and Uhry 1995). As children get a bit older, the Roswell-Chall Auditory Blending Test (Roswell and Chall 1963) can be used effectively to assess their oral sound blending skills; here the examiner says parts of words aloud and the student combines them to form whole words. Full phoneme segmentation, the opposite skill of blending, is often measured by having students use blocks or tiles, without letters, to represent sounds. The Test of Awareness of Language Segments (Sawyer 1987) and the Lindamood Auditory Conceptualization Test (Lindamood and Lindamood 1979) are two commercially available instruments for this.

Measures for older students include the Sound Blending and Incomplete Words subtests of the Woodcock-Johnson Psycho-Educational Battery-Revised (Woodcock and Johnson 1990). The Sound Blending subtest asks students to listen to segmented words and then state them as whole words, while the Incomplete Words subtest requires students to use auditory closure skills to "fill in" the missing segments of dictated words and pronounce them as whole words. Norms on both tests are available through adult levels. The Rosner Test of Auditory Analysis Skills (TAAS; Rosner 1975; Rosner and Simon 1971) is a deletion task in which students from grades K-6 are asked to conceptualize the location of phonemes, delete one, and then blend the others into a new word. The TAAS assumes facility with consonant clusters, which poor readers often find complex and difficult units to segment (Bruck and Treiman 1990). Informal, teacher-developed measures are also likely to provide useful data about students' proficiency in phonological awareness that may be used for assessing dyslexia.

As with the RAN and verbal short-term memory measures, none of the phonological awareness activities should be used in isolation to make instructional decisions. Stanovich (1986) noted that poor decoding is correlated with phonological awareness, not dyslexia. Thus, information about skills in phonological processing must be integrated with discrepancy evidence from other cognitive and academic testing before a decision about the existence of dyslexia can be made.

Inventory of Reading Skills and Strategies

To determine appropriate and effective prescriptive/remedial techniques, clinicians and teachers must inventory students' strengths and weaknesses with regard to reading skills and strategies. By using curriculum-based assessment (CBA) and criterion-referenced instruments, observation, and clinical teaching, they can ascertain which material has been mastered, which skills need reinforcement, and how students might respond to different instructional strategies.

Use of CBA and Criterion-Referenced Instruments. Curriculum-based assessment and criterion-referenced instruments offer opportunities to teachers and clinicians to observe students' oral decoding in connected text (oral reading fluency). Teacher-made tests containing sets of graded reading passages from current instructional materials (CBA) yield information about reading speed and accuracy (King-Sears 1994). Student performances on these measures or on commercial informal reading inventories, such as the Qualitative Reading Inventory-2 (Leslie and Caldwell 1995) or Analytical Reading Inventory (Woods and Moe 1995) help to establish independent, instructional, and frustration reading levels, as well as document strategies and miscues. Observation and taping (video and/or audio) permit clinicians and teachers to ascertain the extent to which students make full use of cue systems (e.g., letters, pictures, contextual meaning, activation of prior knowledge, and use of metacognitive strategies) and whether those cue systems are being integrated or used in isolation (Clark and Uhry 1995; Smith, Goodman, and Meredith 1976).

Other commercial inventories enable practitioners to create profiles of letter names, letter sounds, and sight words mastered. The Brigance Diagnostic Inventory (Brigance 1977) and Roswell and Chall's diagnostic Assessment of Reading (1992) provide methods of collecting and organizing these data. Curriculum-based assessment techniques, reflective of material actually taught in the classroom, are also effective in documenting skill mastery. The profiles may then be used to plan for prescriptive instruction.

Further information about students' phonological awareness and phonics knowledge may be obtained from analysis of their spelling errors on spelling list words and in writing samples. Administration of standardized spelling measures may be followed by use of a phonetically organized list such as the Spellmaster Lists (Greenbaum 1987) to document mastery of basic letter-sound patterns (Clark and Uhry 1995). Students' spelling in writing samples may be weaker and more inconsistent than that on isolated lists because they are easily caught up in the generation of ideas and do not use effective strategies for encoding words whose automatized spellings have not been mastered. Analysis of error patterns may yield prescriptive information for remedial instruction.

Trial Teaching. Trial teaching of potential reading and spelling skills using different approaches can be useful in planning instruction. Exploring possible teaching options can be useful in planning reading and spelling instruction. Practitioners might suggest alternative approaches for decoding or encoding, such as, use of familiar word patterns, breaking words into syllables, or determination of root words and affixes. Students might also be provided with guided instruction in the use of specific strategies for reading or writing (e.g., cloze, graphic organizers) to gauge their potential effectiveness in the classroom.

APPROPRIATE CLASSROOM INTERVENTIONS

While the causes and assessment of dyslexia are debated in the research arena, teachers are struggling with how to accommodate such students in the general education program or how to provide remediation in specialized educational settings. Understanding how normal reading is acquired may be critical to understanding what goes wrong during the development of reading skills in children with dyslexia. Theories about how reading is acquired often influence decisions about what curriculum materials to use.

In the early grades, students learn to read so that by grade three they can begin to use reading to learn specific content. Everything that happens in the classroom revolves around reading. Traditional views on learning to read came from the information processing perspective, where information was taken in at the sensory level, organized and in-

terpreted, stored in short-term memory and categorized for later retrieval (Clark and Uhry 1995). To what extent, then, is reading influenced by the small units of print versus the meaning of the context?

Theories Regarding Acquisition of Reading

Theories about how students acquire reading skills can be organized
into four conceptual models: the top-down processing model (Goodman 1967; Smith 1979), the bottom-up processing model (LeBarge and
Samuels 1994), the interactive model (Rummelhart 1977), and the interactive-compensatory model (Stanovich 1994).

Top-down Processing Model. Theorists subscribing to a top-down
model (Goodman 1967; Smith 1976) emphasize the importance of
meaning in understanding how reading develops. Good readers do
not process every word but select specific knowledge of graphemic,
syntactic, and semantic features of the language needed to construct
meaning from the text. The reader makes informed guesses about the
meaning of a passage based on past experiences and information
gleaned from the text. When those guesses do not make sense, the
reader returns to the text and focuses on specific words and concepts.
This model moves from the cognitive, higher-order thinking skills, to
the sensory or perceptual processes involved in lower order word
identification skills. The implication for instruction, from the beginning, is aimed at the meaning level with limited instruction at the
word or letter level. An example of a curriculum philosophy based on
the top-down model of reading acquisition is a whole language approach (Hollingsworth and Reutzel 1988; Mather 1992); a literature-
based approach such as Reader's Workshop (Atwell 1989); or the
integrated language arts approach to reading. Beliefs about top-down
processing in reading have been called into question by studies which
have demonstrated that good readers do not skip words or phrases. In
fact, Stanovich (1994) has suggested that good readers actually rely
less on the context than do poor readers, who are not so adept at word
recognition and have a slower rate of reading. Accurate and fluent
word recognition is essential for proficient reading. Thus, for reading
disabled students who need direct instruction at the word identification level, research has shown whole word approaches are less effective (Hollingsworth and Reutzel 1988; Mather 1992).

Bottom-up Models. The bottom-up model describes reading as a hierarchy of skills progressing from the smallest bits of graphemic information (letters) to larger chunks of information (words and phrases).
An association is built between low level pieces of information (sound

and symbol) and is then interpreted and associated with specific meanings. Essential to this model is the necessity for skills to become automatic so that reading becomes fluent. LeBerge and Samuels (1974) explain the need for the many components of reading to be coordinated in a short time, automatically, so that sufficient energy and attention are available for comprehension. Classroom implications for this model are obvious: letters and sounds must be taught before words, words before sentences, and sentences before passages. This model is the basis for most basal reading programs used in elementary schools. More specifically, remedial approaches based on the Orton-Gillingham approach (Gillingham and Stillman 1969; Orton 1966) of teaching reading follow this model. This will be discussed in more depth later.

Interactive Models. Clark and Uhry (1995) describe the difference between top-down, bottom-up, and interactive models by contrasting the serial nature of top-down and bottom-up models with the parallel nature of the interactive model.

> In both models [top-down and bottom-up] control over the reading process operates in one direction; each processing event triggers another processing event, either one step up or one step down in a hierarchy. In contrast, another view of reading holds that many of the component processes occur at the same time or in parallel. (p. 7)

Associations between word identification in context and prediction of meaning occur simultaneously. Proficient readers use multiple sources of information, some related to the grapheme-phoneme relationship, others to the semantic aspect of the text. Additionally, metacognitive knowledge, as well as background information, contributes to the overall comprehension of the text.

Such connections, Clark and Urhy explain, happen "all at once rather than in a linear, hierarchical fashion" (p. 8). Such a model has received support from Stanovich (1984) in his Interactive-Compensatory Model of Reading, in which he describes a confluence of developmental, experimental, and educational psychology. In addition to the idea that "recognition takes place via the simultaneous amalgamation of information from many different knowledge sources" (p. 15), Stanovich adds a compensatory assumption "that deficiencies at any level in the processing hierarchy can be compensated for by a greater use of information from other levels" (p. 15). Effective classroom instruction based on such a model includes strong elements of a whole language, meaning-based approach with systematic, direct instruction in phonics.

"The Great Debate" as described by Chall (1983) highlights the current situation. Should reading instruction in the general classroom be phonics based or meaning based? As methods of instruction designed to help students with dyslexia are examined, it is important to remember that a significant number of these students are in the general education classroom with little or no support from specialists in reading. These students are often lost along the continuum, as the pendulum swings back and forth between whole language philosophies and direct instruction methods. As discussed earlier, if dyslexia is viewed primarily as a language-based deficit, the implications for classroom instruction become clear.

Predicting later reading success from an early language processing ability has been shown to have a significant relationship. Promising work by Tallal and Merzenich (1996) in the area of training programs for language learning-impaired children may provide the necessary basis for improvements in phonological and grammatical analyses as well as for other language data; however, gains that transfer to the acquisition of reading skills have not been demonstrated.

According to Catts (1989), there are possibly two groups of children with reading deficits: those whose global language impairment causes later reading impairment and those whose dyslexia affects only specific areas of language development. Specific deficits in phonological processing include speech perception, verbal short-term memory, speech articulation rate, rapid naming, and phonological awareness deficits. In addition to these "core phonological" deficits are other factors, such as attention deficits, which are of equal importance to classroom intervention and often confuse the issue of what is causing the reading disability (Felton and Woods 1989).

Classroom Manifestation of Dyslexia

How does dyslexia manifest itself in the classroom? Certainly as a word-reading disorder, but also with related problems in spelling, phonological processing, reading rate, comprehension, handwriting, and written expression. The most pronounced difficulty these students have is the inability to decode unfamiliar words. Although the reasons for this are debated among researchers and clinicians, classroom teachers must (a) address the deficit in the ability to use sound/symbol associations and understand similarities and differences in sound structures and (b) do so with twenty-five other students in the class.

For some students with dyslexia, word recognition may be a strength when these words are presented in context. Teachers must use this ability when developing strategies for strengthening weak decoding skills. A slow rate of reading has also been found to be a significant problem (Perfetti and Hogaboam 1975). The Colorado Reading Project (Defries et al. 1991) has been looking at this aspect of reading disorder and has found that even with improved word recognition and decoding, a slow rate of reading continues to be a problem greatly affecting comprehension.

Many programs have targeted one or more aspects of reading disability. Some work well in large group settings, such as the general classroom, while others require a small group or one-to-one tutorial approach. Specialized techniques such as the Orton-Gillingham approach (Gillingham and Stillman 1960) emphasize direct instruction in phonics while other programs such as Auditory Discrimination in Depth (Lindamood and Lindamood 1975) develop phonological awareness. Both, however, require intensive amounts of one-to-one time with students, which simply may not be available in the general education classroom. The implications from this are particularly relevant in today's climate of full inclusion for all students.

Direct Instruction. One of the most often acknowledged principles applied to remedial intervention is direct instruction. This direct, intensive, and systematic work is important for students with dyslexia (Bryant 1980) and should be carried out by highly trained professionals, not parent volunteers or teacher aides. Three models of direct instruction have been used: a tutoring model (Traub 1982); a small group model (Cox 1955; Enfield and Green 1981); and a whole class model (Wolf 1985). Whichever model is employed by teachers, it should be remembered that students with dyslexia will require more time in direct instruction than other students. In a group model, many students with dyslexia become overloaded by the pace of instruction. Four factors contributing to this overload are: slow speed of processing, difficulty automatizing information learned, failure to apply strategies, and distractibility (Bryant 1980). Few available reading methods deal with all these factors and, thus, teachers need to choose and combine aspects of many approaches when building comprehensive classroom instruction.

Learning to Mastery. Gaining automaticity is critical to mastery learning. As LeBerge and Samuels (1974) indicate, automatic processing at the word level frees up working memory to allow more efficient processing at the sentence and passage levels. Prompting techniques decrease the possibility of errors while helping students respond. In addition, demonstration, guided practice, response, and independent practice are essential. Monitoring and evaluation through curriculum-based assessment and daily record keeping become critical components to successful treatment.

Multisensory Learning. As early as the 1940s, interventions used a multisensory approach. Grace Fernald (1943) first introduced the visual-auditory-kinesthetic-tactile (or VAKT method), in which students used sensory channels such as tactile (touch) and kinesthesis (movement) to support or enhance the visual and auditory input to produce a memory schema for words. During the 1960s, Gillingham and Stillman combined these multisensory techniques with the teachings of Dr. Samuel Orton to develop the Orton-Gillingham approach, the basis for many programs designed to help students use kinesthetic activities to establish visual-auditory associations in letter-sound correspondence.

Remediating Dyslexia

Instruction aimed at remediating dyslexia must focus on those deficits known to be associated with reading disability while building on the strengths available in each student. Direct instruction in phonics, training in phonological awareness, techniques for improving reading comprehension, programs for expanding language and background knowledge, as well as metacognitive strategies and computer-assisted instruction are all available as tools for classroom teachers in designing relevant instruction.

Phonics Instruction and Phonological Awareness. Both phonics and phonological awareness are important components of sound reading instruction, but they are not the same thing. Clark and Urhy explain the difference this way:

> Phonics is defined here as low level rote knowledge of the association between letters and sounds. . . . Phonological awareness includes a range of higher level metacognitive understanding of word boundaries within spoken sentences, of syllable boundaries in spoken words, and of how to isolate phonemes and establish their location within syllables and words. (p. 75)

Most explicit phonics training programs do not include specific training in phonological awareness. Specific training in phonological awareness has been done at three levels: prereading (Rosner 1974; Venezky 1976); beginning reading (Blackman 1987); and remedial reading (Lindamood 1994; Torgesen 1995; Williams 1980).

Explicit phonics programs teach individual grapheme-phoneme correspondences before they are blended to form syllables and words. Examples of such programs are the Orton-Gillingham approach (Gillingham and Stillman 1960); Alphabetic Phonics (Cox 1985); Recipe for Reading (Traub and Bloom 1975); and the Wilson Reading

System (Wilson 1988). Each of these methods requires specific teacher training that exceeds pre-service college preparation. Information about training is available through many sources, from universities to special interest groups such as The International Dyslexia Association.

Instructional Programs Using A Phonics Approach. The Orton-Gillingham approach (Gillingham and Stillman 1960) is designed for one-to-one instruction. It is a direct approach to the study of phonics, presenting the sounds of the phonograms orally as separate units and teaching the process of blending them, first into syllables and then into words. It is an integrated total language approach using visual, auditory, and kinesthetic components to reinforce learning. It is systematic as it proceeds from simple to complex structures in an orderly progression of language development. In the Orton-Gillingham approach, reading of text begins only when the student is able to read c-v-c (consonant-vowel-consonant) words perfectly and automatically, as well as phonetic four-letter words with digraphs such as *th* and *ph*. Text reading begins with words the student has learned with nonphonetic words the student does not know, underlined, so that the teacher can tell them to the student. Written language is taught along with direct instruction so that a knowledge of spelling patterns can be given to the students. Teachers can use commercially available books, such as linguistic readers to supplement instruction.

Alphabetic Phonics (Cox 1988) is an organization and expansion of the Orton-Gillingham multisensory approach and was developed by Aylette Cox (1985). It is also designed for one-to-one instruction, based on the premise that 80% of the most commonly used English words can be considered phonetically regular and, therefore, predictable once certain rules have been learned. Progress is documented through the use of Benchmark Measures coordinated with the schedules or steps in the sequenced program. As its name implies, Alphabetic Phonics stresses the unique characteristics of written English. The structured daily lesson takes an hour to complete, with eleven activities typically lasting from three to ten minutes each, including language orientation, sequence and directionality of the alphabet, reading and spelling decks, reading phonetically controlled text, handwriting, and listening.

Recipe for Reading, developed by Nina Traub (1975), is another adaptation of the Gillingham approach. It applies a synthetic phonics approach, teaching individual letter sounds in isolation before introducing syllables and words. Teaching follows a part-to-whole progression, designed for grades one through three. It should be delivered on a one-to-one basis outside the classroom in half hour sessions, five days a week.

The Wilson Reading System (Wilson 1988) is one of the few remedial programs developed specifically for adults and adolescents with dyslexia. It, too, is based on the Orton-Gillingham principles and is a multisensory, synthetic approach to teaching reading and writing. Wilson believes that many older students have developed a block to reading because they have come to think of printed English as so lacking in regularity that it is impossible to learn. One-to-one tutoring is the ideal setting; however, it has been used successfully with small groups of students in school settings. The program is sequenced in twelve steps based on six syllable types, one innovation that Wilson brings to the Orton-Gillingham program.

Phoneme awareness is the ability to analyze and manipulate sounds within syllables: to count, delete, and reorder them. Auditory Discrimination in Depth (ADD) was developed by Charles and Pat Lindamood (1975) as a preventive, developmental, or remedial program designed to teach auditory conceptualization skills basic to reading, spelling, and speech. It can be used with prereaders or beginning readers to bolster their development of auditory-perceptual awareness, or with older children or adults who fail to read and spell successfully because of a failure to acquire phonemic analysis skills. Auditory Discrimination in Depth requires specific training to implement the program, which contains five developmental levels beginning with auditory perception, identifying and classifying speech sounds, distinguishing and naming the various sound categories, spelling activities using real words, and finally reading text. During the second level, students are taught to categorize and label on the basis of shape and position of the lips, teeth, and tongue when sounds are produced. It is during this stage that students learn about "lip poppers" (b and p) and "tip tappers" (t and d). Providing an articulatory foundation for identifying phoneme segments is important since children with dyslexia are deficient in several basic phonological processes.

An extension of auditory discrimination in depth, the Reading with Orthographic and Segmented Speech (ROSS) program, uses talking computers to remediate deficits in word recognition and phonological awareness. When reading stories on a screen, children can request assistance with any words they do not know. The program then highlights the word in segments and pronounces the segments in order.

Another computerized remediation has been developed by Tallal and associates (1996). These computer generated audio-visual games are designed to train language-learning impaired children in temporal processing. Tallal suggests that some language learning impairment may relate to a defective representation of speech phonetics, embedded through learning, that can be overcome with specific training in temporal processing. How such training will translate into gains in reading remains an area to be researched.

Project Read (Enfield and Greene 1969) began as a three-year experimental program to deliver direct, systematic phonics instruction in regular classrooms to students performing below the 25th percentile in reading and spelling. It was designed as a cost effective reading instruction program to coordinate regular classroom instruction with remedial instruction while keeping students "in the mainstream." It is now used in classrooms and resource rooms with students from elementary through secondary levels. The curriculum is composed of three phases: instruction in phonics, reading comprehension, and written expression. Phase I, phonics, is essentially a modification of the Orton-Gillingham approach, providing a systematic sequence of skills and oral reading using a basic linguistic reading series. Phase II focuses on reading comprehension and vocabulary development, while Phase III encompasses written expression.

The Direct Instruction Model, which became known as DISTAR, was developed by Becker and Engelmann (1968) for use with educational programs for disadvantaged children in the first three grades. Building on a strong belief in teaching basic skills, the program aims to "even the playing field" for disadvantaged children. However, DISTAR has been used to teach children with a variety of learning disabilities. It provides a rapid-paced, teacher-directed, small-group instructional model with continuous positive reinforcement and biweekly progress monitoring. All instruction follows a script providing exact wording and precise directions for teachers. The program has three levels: Level One builds vocabulary, develops oral language skills, and establishes the foundation for logical thinking; Level 2 builds a language foundation for reading comprehension; and Level 3 focuses on reading mastery.

Metacognitive Approaches to Remediating Reading Problems. There are other approaches that focus on the metacognitive strategies for both decoding and comprehension. Such approaches rely heavily on the students' abilities to learn how and when to apply a specific problem-solving strategy.

Project READ, developed by Robert Calfee and associates (1985), has as its central goal, competence in applying language as a tool for thinking and communication. Four instructional propositions underlie the program. The first is simplicity. Complex tasks should be broken down into relatively coherent subtasks. The second is that language skills are interrelated and should be taught as such. The third principle is that teaching the formal use of language is the most important goal of schooling; and the fourth proposition is that direct teaching (combined with small group discussion) is essential to effective reading instruction. The curriculum focuses on decoding, vocabulary development, comprehension of narrative text, and comprehension of expository text. It was designed for use with a basal reading series, but has been adapted for use with literature-based curricula as well.

Strategy-based instructional approaches such as the ones developed at the University of Kansas (Deshler and Schumaker 1986) are designed to provide auditory and graphic organizers to structure problem solving. Each strategy is a tool for facilitating learning and must be evaluated for its effectiveness and efficiency for each student and the task at hand. The instructional environment must be modified to promote strategy use with each strategy containing a set of sequential steps that lead to a specific outcome and successful completion of the task. The steps should cue selection and use of appropriate procedures, rules, and skills. Specific strategies for reading have been developed to address writing skills (TRIMS), word identification and paraphrasing, error monitoring (PENS and COPS), and comprehension.

Improving the thinking skills of students is at the heart of techniques developed by McTighe and Lyman (1988). These strategies bring sound instructional theory into the classroom in a practical form that both students and teachers enjoy using. Think-Pair-Share, the Thinking Matrix, Reading Reference, and Cognitive Mapping (McTighe and Lyman 1988) are all tools teachers can use to apply a metacognitive approach to reading instruction. These tools serve as catalysts for creating a responsive "thinking" classroom. They aid memory, provide a common frame of reference and incentive to act, together with a framework for permanent application of innovative teaching. These tools are concrete, and remind teachers and students to use what they already know to enhance learning. The use of graphic organizers to represent thinking also provides teachers and students with visual representations of the metacognitive strategy required. These graphic organizers are particularly useful in improving reading comprehension.

Reciprocal Teaching, developed by Palincsar and Brown (1985), is another technique useful in improving reading comprehension. During this activity, teachers and students take turns assuming the roles of teacher and lead dialogue sessions about the passages read. All the participants share common goals of predicting, question generation, summarizing, and clarifying. Teachers explain what strategies will be learned, why, and when to apply them. Then they model each strategy, allowing students to summarize and add their own predictions, clarifications, and responses to questions. Through guided practice, responsibility for leading the dialogue is gradually transferred to the students. This type of cooperative learning activity helps students use their prior knowledge in mastering new content information.

Many cooperative learning strategies have been developed. One such program, Cooperative Integrated Reading and Composition (CIRC) (Slavin, Stevens, and Madden 1988) applies the principles of cooperative learning to other research in reading, writing, spelling, and English mechanics. Students are divided into reading levels and then assigned to teams of four or five students each. They are then paired so that they have partners on their reading levels. Using basal readers, students work in teams to gain mastery of vocabulary, decoding, and content. In addition to the teamwork, there is also time for independent silent reading. Lessons are teacher-directed, with follow-up activities completed in the team areas. CIRC has been demonstrated to be a useful tool when students with reading disabilities are included in general education settings.

Integrating Technology into the Reading Program.   Teachers are beginning to use available technology in the classroom. During the "Learning to Read" stage, technology can provide supplemental drill and practice as well as direct instruction or training in phonics and phonological awareness (Torgesen and Young 1984). During this period of skill acquisition, students can use computers to extend direct instruction ordinarily provided by their teachers. To be used effectively, however, teachers must go beyond this drill and practice stage and begin to incorporate technology into the "Reading to Learn" stage as well. Excellent software exists that allows students to expand their concept development, vocabulary, and problem-solving skills. Remedial educators must collaborate with general education teachers to adapt available software for use by students with dyslexia. One example of such software is the laser disk technology that encourages the application of reading skills through cooperative learning activities in the content areas of science and social studies.

Finally, teachers must begin to utilize the vast amount of information available to students over the Internet. Using technology, students with dyslexia, who have great difficulty with higher-level expressive writing, can now put together multimedia presentations that far surpass any previously written work.

The challenges of teaching students with dyslexia in today's world may seem overwhelming to teachers expected to meet the needs of all learners in general education classrooms. However, instruction in small group situations and even one-to-one instruction in more restricted settings must remain options, available to educators and students alike, if the challenge of remediating reading disabilities is to be met and conquered.

REFERENCES

Adams, M. J., and Bruck, M. 1995. Resolving the great debate. *American Educator* 19: 7–12.

Adams, M. J. 1990. *Beginning to Read: Thinking and Learning About Print.* Cambridge, MA: MIT Press.

Atwell, N. 1989. *In the Middle: Writing, Reading, and Learning with Adolescents.* Portsmouth, NH: Boynton/Cook.

Beck, I. L., and Juel, C. 1995. The role of decoding in learning to read. *American Educator* 19: 8–12.

Berk, R. A. 1982. Effectiveness of discrepancy score methods for screening children with learning disabilities. *Learning Disabilities* 1:11–24.

Berk, R. A. 1984 . *Screening and Diagnosis of Children with Learning Disabilities.* Springfield, IL: Charles C Thomas.

Blachman, B. 1987. An alternative classroom reading program for learning disabled and other low-achieving children. In *Intimacy with Language: A Forgotten Basic in Teacher Education*, ed. R. Bowler. Baltimore: The Orton Dyslexia Society.

Brigance, A. 1977. *Brigance Diagnostic Inventory of Basic Skills.* North Billerica, MA: Curriculum Associates.

Brown, R. T., and Modan-Swain, A. 1993. Cognitive neuropsychological and academic sequelae in children with leukemia. *Journal of Learning Disabilities* 26:74–90.

Bruck, M., and Treiman, R. 1990. Phonological awareness and spelling in normal children and dyslexics: The case of initial consonant clusters. *Journal of Experimental Child Psychology* 50:156–78.

Bryant, N. D., Canale, F., Driscoll, R., Fayne, H., Fisher, J., Gettinger, M., Gluckman, J., Kowalski, L., Rovinski, N., and Tardis, V. 1979. *The Effects of Instructional Variables on the Learning of Handicapped and Non-Handicapped Individuals. Research Review Series, Vol. 1.* New York: Columbia University Teachers College Research Institute for the Study of Learning Disabilities.

Calfee, R., and Henry, M. 1985. Project READ: An inservice model for training classroom teachers in effective reading instruction. In *The Effective Teaching of Reading: Theory, and Practice*, ed. J. Hoffman. Newark, DE: International Reading Association.

Catts, H. W. 1991. Early identification of dyslexia: Evidence from a follow-up study of speech-language impaired children. *Annals of Dyslexia* 41:163–177.

Chall, J. S. 1983. *Learning to Read: The Great Debate.* New York: McGraw-Hill.

Clark, D. B., and Uhry, J. K. 1995. *Dyslexia: Theory and Practice of Remedial Instruction* (2nd edition). Baltimore, MD: York Press.

Cox, B. A. 1985. Alphabetic phonics: An organization and expansion of Orton-Gillingham. *Annals of Dyslexia* 35:187–98.

DeFries, J. C., Olson, R. K., Pennington, B. F., and Smith, S. D. 1991. Colorado reading project: An update. In *The Reading Brain: The Biological Basis of Dyslexia*, eds. D. Duane and D. Gray. Parkton, MD: York Press.

Denckla, M. B., and Rudel, R. G. 1974. Rapid automatized naming of pictured objects, colors, letters, and numbers by normal children. *Cortex* 10:186–202.

Deshler, D. D., and Schumaker, J. B. 1986. Learning strategies: An instructional alternative for low-achieving adolescents. *Exceptional Children* 52(6): 583–90.

Enfield, M. L, and Greene, V. E. 1981. There is a skeleton in every closet. *Bulletin of The Orton Society* 31:189–98.

Fawcett, A. J., and Nicolson, R. I. 1994. Naming speed in children with dyslexia. *Journal of Learning Disabilities* 27:641–46.

Felton, R. H., and Wood, F. B. 1989. Cognitive deficits in reading disability and attention deficit disorder. *Journal of Learning Disabilities* 22:3–22.

Fernald, G. M. 1943. *Remedial Techniques in Basic School Subjects*. New York: McGraw-Hill.

Fletcher, J. M., and Loveland, K. A. 1986. Neuropsychology of arithmetic disabilities in children. *Focus on Learning Problems in Mathematics* 8:23–40.

Fletcher, J. M. 1992. The validity of distinguishing children with language and learning disabilities according to discrepancies with IQ: Introduction to the special series. *Journal of Learning Disabilities* 25:546–48.

Fletcher, J. M., Shaywitz, S. E., Shankweiler, D., Katz, L., Liberman, I. Y., Steubing, K. K., Francis, D. J., Fowler, A. F., and Shaywitz, B. A. 1994. Cognitive profiles of reading disability: Comparisons of discrepancy and low achievement definitions. *Journal of Educational Psychology* 86:6–23.

Gillingham, A., and Stillman, B. 1973. *Remedial Training for Children with Specific Disabilities in Reading, Spelling and Penmanship*. Cambridge, MA: Educators Publishing Service.

Glaser, C. W. 1996. Impacts of multimedia anchored instruction on classroom interaction. Paper presented at the International Learning Disability Association of America. Houston, TX.

Goodman, K. 1967. Reading: A psycholinguistic guessing game. *Journal of the Reading Specialist* 6:126–35.

Gough, P. B., and Tunmer, W. E. 1986. Decoding, reading, and reading disability. *Remedial and Special Education* 7:6–10. Austin, TX: PRO-ED.

Greenbaum, C. R. 1987. *Spellmaster Assessment and Teaching System*. Austin, TX: PRO-ED.

Hammill, D. 1991. *Detroit Tests of Learning Aptitude-Third Edition*. Austin, TX: PRO-ED.

Hill, J. R. 1981. *Measurement and Evaluation in the Classroom*. Columbus, OH: Merrill.

Hollingsworth, P. M., and Reutzel, D. R. 1988. Whole language with LD children. *Academic Therapy* 23(5):477–87.

Johnson, D. J., and Croasmun, P. A. 1991. Language assessment. In *Handbook on the Assessment of Learning Disabilities: Theory, Research, and Practice*, ed. H. L. Swanson. Austin, TX: PRO-ED.

Jorm, A. 1983. Specific reading retardation and working memory: A review. *British Journal of Psychology* 74:311–42.

King-Sears, M. E. 1994. *Curriculum-based Assessment in Special Education*. San Diego, CA: Singular Publishing Group, Inc.

Le Barge, D., and Samuels, S. J. 1974. Toward a theory of automatic information processing reading. *Cognitive Psychology* 6:293–323.

Leslie, L., and Caldwell, J. 1995. *Qualitative Reading Inventory-2*. New York: HarperCollins Publishers.

Lindamood, C. H., and Lindamood, P. C. 1979. *The LAC Test: Lindamood Auditory Conceptualization Test*. Chicago: Riverside.

Lindamood, C. H., and Lindamood, P. C. 1975. *The ADD Program, Auditory Discrimination in Depth*: Books 1 and 2. Austin, TX: PRO-ED.

Lindamood, P. C. 1994. Issues in researching the link between phonological awareness, learning disabilities, and spelling. In *Frames of Reference for the Assessment of Learning Disabilities*, ed. G.R. Lyon. Baltimore, MD: Brookes.

Lyon, G. R. 1995. Toward a definition of dyslexia. *Annals of Dyslexia* XLV: 3–27.

Mather, N. 1992. Whole language reading instruction for students with learning disabilities: Caught in the crossfire. *Learning Disabilities Research & Practice* 7(2):87–95.

McTighe, J., and Lyman, F. T., Jr. 1988. Cueing thinking in the classroom: The promise of theory-embedded tools. *Educational Leadership* 4:18–24.

Merzenich, M. M., Jenkins, W. M., Johnston, P., Schreiner, C., Miller, S. L., and Tallal, P. 1996. Temporal processing deficits of language learning impaired children ameliorated by training. *Science* 271:77–81.

Moats, L. C. 1994. Assessment of spelling. In *Frames of Reference for the Assessment of Learning Disabilities*, ed. G. R. Lyon. Baltimore, MD: Brookes.

Olson, R. K., Conners, F. A., and Rack, J. 1994. Eye movements in normal and dyslexia readers. In *Vision and Visual Dyslexia*, ed. J. F. Stein. London: Macmillan.

Olson, R. K., Forsberg, H., Wise, B., and Rack, J. 1994. Measurement of word recognition, orthographic, and phonological skills. In *Frames of Reference for the Assessment of Learning Disabilities*, ed. G. R. Lyon. Baltimore, MD: Brookes.

Olson, R. K., Wise, B., Conners, F., and Rack, J. P., 1990. Organization, heritability, and remediation of component word recognition and language skills in disabled readers. In *Reading and Its Development: Component Skills Approaches*, eds. T. H. Carr and B. A. Levy. New York: Academic Press.

Olson, R. K., Wise, B., Conners, F., Rack, J. P., and Fulker, D. 1989. Specific deficits in component reading and language skills: Genetic and environmental influences. *Journal of Learning Disabilities*, 22:339–48.

Orton, S. T. 1966. The Orton-Gillingham approach. In *The Disabled Reader*, ed. J. Money. Baltimore: The Johns Hopkins University Press.

Palinscar, A. S., and Brown, A. L. 1988. Teaching and practicing thinking skills to promote comprehension in the context of group problem solving. *Remedial and Special Education* 9(1):53–59.

Pennington, B. F. 1995. Genetics of learning disabilities. *Journal of Child Neurology* 10:69–77.

Perfetti, C. A., and Roth, S. 1981. Some of the interactive processes in reading and their role in reading skill. In *Interactive Processes in Reading*, eds. A. M. Lesgold and C. A. Perfetti. Hillsdale, NJ: Lawrence Erlbaum Associates.

Rack, J. P., Snowling, M. J., and Olson, R. K. 1992. The nonword reading deficit in developmental dyslexia: A review. *Reading Research Quarterly* 27:28–53.

Richardson, E., and DiBenedetto, B. 1985. *Decoding Skills Test.* Los Angeles, CA: Western Psychological Services.

Rosner, J., and Simon, D. P. 1971. The auditory analysis test: An initial report. *Journal of Learning Disabilities* 4:384–92.

Rosner, J. 1975. Test of auditory analysis skills. In *Helping Children Overcome Learning Difficulties.* New York: Walker & Co.

Roswell, F. G., and Chall, J. S. 1963. *Roswell-Chall Auditory Blending Test.* San Diego, CA: Essay Press.

Roswell, F. G., and Chall, J. S. 1992. *Diagnostic Assessment of Reading.* Chicago: Riverside Publishing Co.

Sawyer, D. J. 1987. *Test of Awareness of Language Segments.* Austin, TX: PRO-ED.

Shankweiler, D., and Liberman, I. Y. 1989. *Phonology and Reading Disability.* Ann Arbor, MI: The University of Michigan Press.

Shankweiler, D., Crain, S., Katz, L., Fowler, A. E., Liberman, A., Brady, S. A., Thornton, R., Lundquist, E., Dreyer, L., Fletcher, J. M., Steubing, K. K., Shaywitz, S. E., and Shaywitz, B. A. 1995. Cognitive profiles of reading-disabled children: Comparison of language skills in phonology, morphology, and syntax. *Psychological Science* 6:149–56.

Shaywitz, S. E, Escobar, M. D., Shaywitz, B. A., Fletcher, J. M., and Makuch, R. 1992. Evidence that dyslexia may represent the lower tail of a normal distribution of reading ability. *New England Journal of Medicine* 326:145–50.

Siegel, L. S. 1989. IQ is irrelevant to the definition of learning disabilities. *Journal of Learning Disabilities* 22:469–78.

Slavin, R. E., Stevens, R. J., and Madden, N. A. 1988. Accommodating student diversity in reading and writing instruction: A cooperative learning approach. *Remedial and Special Education* 9(1):60–66.

Smith, E. B., Goodman, K. S., and Meredith, R. 1976. *Language and Thinking in School.* 2nd ed. New York: Rinehart & Winston.

Smith, F. 1979. Conflicting approaches to reading research and instruction. In *Theory and Practice of Early Reading*: Vol. 2, eds. L. B. Resnick and P.A. Weaver. Hillsdale, N.J.: Lawrence Erlbaum Associates.

Stanovich, K. E., and Siegel, L. S. 1994. Phenotypic performance profile of children with reading disabilities: A regression-based test of the phonological-core variable-difference model. *Journal of Educational Psychology* 86:24–53.

Stanovich, K. E. 1984. The interactive-compensatory model of reading: A confluence of developmental, experimental, and educational psychology. *Remedial and Special Education* 5:11–19.

Stanovich, K. E. 1986. Matthew effects in reading: Some consequences of individual differences in the acquisition of literacy. *Reading Research Quarterly* 21: 7–29.

Stanovich, K. E. 1988. Explaining the difference between the dyslexic and the garden-variety poor reader: The phonological-core variable-difference model. *Journal of Learning Disabilities* 21:590–604.

Stanovich, K. E. 1990. Concepts in developmental theories of reading skill: Cognitive resources, automaticity, modularity. *Developmental Review* 19:72–100.

Stanovich, K. E. 1991a. Discrepancy definitions of reading disability: Has intelligence led us astray? *Reading Research Quarterly* 26:7–29.

Stanovich, K. E. 1991b. Reading disability: Assessment issues. In *Handbook on the Assessment of Learning Disabilities: Theory, Research, and Practice,* ed. H. L. Swanson. Austin, TX: PRO-ED.

Stark, R. E., Bernstein, L. E., Condino, R., Bender, M., Tallal, P., and Catts, H. 1984. Four-year follow-up study of language impaired children. *Annals of Dyslexia* 34:49–68.

Swanson, H. L. 1996. *Swanson Cognitive Processing Test.* Austin, TX: PRO-ED.

Tallal, P., Miller, S. L., Bedi, G., Byma, G., Wang, X., Nagarajan, S. S., Schreiner, C., Jenkins, W. M., and Merzenich, M. M. 1996. Language comprehension in language-learning impaired children improved with acoustically modified speech. *Science* 271:81–84.

Torgesen, J. K., and Young, K. A. 1984. Priorities for the use of microcomputer with learning disabled children. *Annual Review of Learning Disabilities* 2: 143–46.

Torgesen, J. K., and Bryant, B. R. 1994. *Test of Phonological Awareness.* Austin, TX: PRO-ED.

Traub, N., and Bloom, F. 1975. *Recipe for Reading.* Cambridge, MA: Educators Publishing Service.

Venezky, R. L. 1976. Prerequisites for learning to read. In *Cognitive Learning in Children: Theories and Strategies,* eds. R. Levin and V. L. Allen. New York: Academic Press.

Wechsler, D. 1991. *Wechsler Individual Achievement Test.* San Antonio, TX: The Psychological Corporation.

Wechsler, D. 1991. *Wechsler Intelligence Scale for Children-Third Edition.* San Antonio, TX: The Psychological Corporation.

Wechsler, D. 1992. *Wechsler Individual Achievement Test.* San Antonio, TX: The Psychological Corporation.

Williams, J. B. 1980. Teaching decoding with an emphaisis on phoneme analysis and phoneme blending. *Journal of Eduational Psychology* 72:1–15.

Wilson, B. A. 1988. *Wilson Reading System Program Overview.* Millbury, MA: Wilson Language Training.

Wood, F., Felton, R., Flowers, L., and Naylor, C. 1991. Neurobehavioral definition of dyslexia. In *The Reading Brain: The Biological Basis of Dyslexia,* eds. D. D. Duane and D. B. Gray. Parkton, MD: York Press.

Woodcock R., and Johnson, M. B. 1990. *Woodcock-Johnson Psycho-Educational Battery-Revised.* Chicago: Riverside.

Woods, M. L., and Moe, A. J. 1995. *Analytic Reading Inventory.* Columbus, OH: Merrill.

Chapter • 10

Instructional Interventions for Children with Reading Disabilities

Joseph K. Torgesen

Perhaps no other topic in the history of education has been the subject of such heated discussion and controversy as the issue of how we should teach young children to read. There have been an enormous number of research studies on this topic (Adams 1990; Clark 1988), but this research has not produced a strong consensus: there are still many differences of opinion among both researchers and teachers on this issue. Part of the problem, of course, is that the question of how best to teach children to read is too broad to be addressed by a single answer. Answers to this question will depend on many factors, such as the skills and attitudes that children bring with them to school, the skills, personality, and motivation of their teachers, and the support provided to children in their homes and neighborhoods. With this range of factors affecting children's responses to instruction, it is not too surprising that we do not have a stronger consensus about which instructional methods are most appropriate for children who experience difficulties learning to read.

Although there are no simple ways around the difficulties of obtaining clear, widely applicable research answers to questions about instruction for children with reading disabilities, several recent advances in the scientific study of reading and reading disabilities do make it possible to conduct studies that may lead to more definitive answers than have been available in the past. In this chapter, I will review some of our recently acquired knowledge about reading and reading disabilities that provides a context for modern research on intervention. Following this introductory overview, I will present preliminary results from two intervention projects we have been conducting over the last several years, and I will conclude with some general comments summarizing current knowledge about effective interventions for children with reading disabilities.

RECENT ADVANCES IN KNOWLEDGE ABOUT READING AND READING DISABILITIES

The last 20 years have been extremely productive for the scientific study of reading and reading disabilities. We now have a much improved understanding of the nature and developmental course of specific developmental reading disability (dyslexia), and we also have acquired significant new knowledge about the reading acquisition process per se. In order to provide a context for these new findings, I will first make a few general points about reading that are not new, and on which there should be fairly widespread agreement among both researchers and practitioners.

General Facts About Reading Ability and Reading Instruction

The first point is that the ultimate goal of all reading instruction is to help children acquire the skills they need to comprehend written materials at a level consistent with their general ability and knowledge. We also want children to enjoy reading so that they will read on their own. Reading is a skill whose ultimate purpose is to help children and adults obtain learning and enjoyment through understanding printed material.

It is also widely known that two broadly different kinds of skills are required to support good reading comprehension. The first set of skills are those required for identifying the printed words on the page (Beck and Juel 1995). This set of skills must be acquired to make the translation between oral and written language. As they increase their word reading skills, children eventually learn several different ways to identify words. They will learn how to use letter-sound correspondences to "sound out" words, and they will also come to recognize very large numbers of words, immediately, as whole units. Other words might be read by analogy to known words, such as when the child gets a start in reading the word "cannon" by recognizing that the first part of the word is already known as "can." Finally, children will also become adept at using the meaningful context of a passage to help them constrain their search for a word's identity.

As we shall see later, the use of grapheme-phoneme correspondences or phonetic decoding, the use of analogy, and dependence on context for help in identifying words are more characteristic of children as they are learning to read. Skillful readers read most of the words in text very rapidly in a single glance, which is sometimes referred to as "sight word reading" (Ehri in press).

Another important set of skills that contribute to good reading comprehension are those that are involved in constructing the meaning of the text. Knowledge of word meanings, or vocabulary, is of critical importance here (Beck and McKeown 1991). Also important is one's general knowledge of the subject matter referred to in the text. It is easier for most people to comprehend written material about local politics than about atomic physics! As children read different forms of text, they become familiar with print conventions, such as the organizing or introductory function of the first sentence in a paragraph, which also aids comprehension. Various thinking skills, such as reasoning and inference making are also required in order to construct accurately the meaning of text. Finally, many different cognitive strategies can be used to enhance comprehension, or repair it when it breaks down (Palincsar and Brown 1984). For example, one commonly taught strategy is for children to monitor their comprehension consistently by asking themselves questions about what they are reading, and then to reread if they discover a lapse in their understanding.

If one considers the skills required to construct the meaning of text, it is clear they overlap to a large extent with those required for oral language comprehension. Phil Gough and his colleagues (Gough 1996; Gough and Hillinger 1980) have proposed what they refer to as "the simple view" of reading to describe the way word identification (decoding) skills and language comprehension skills interact with one another to produce reading comprehension. According to Gough (1996) ". . . reading consists of two parts. One is recognizing the words on the page, the other is understanding those words once you have recognized them. We have called this the Simple View of reading. According to the Simple View, reading equals the product of decoding (D) and comprehension (C), or R = D X C" (p. 4).

Although this simple formula may not capture some of the subtle interactions between decoding and comprehension processes during reading, it does do a very good empirical job of describing how these two broadly different kinds of skills combine to produce good reading comprehension. That is, if one independently measures decoding, or word reading skills, and listening comprehension skills, and then multiplies them together, the resulting product correlates about .84 to .91 (from first through fourth grades) with measured reading comprehension (Hoover and Gough 1990). All this suggests is that both types of skills are essential for good reading comprehension. It is difficult to comprehend the meaning of a text in which many of the words are not accurately identified. Likewise, limited knowledge of a subject, or lack of understanding of many of the words in a text will limit one's comprehension no matter how accurately the specific words are pronounced.

What Aspects of Reading are Particularly Difficult for Children with Dyslexia?

Having identified two broadly different kinds of skills required for good reading comprehension, it seems appropriate to ask if children with reading disabilities find one or another of these skills particularly difficult to acquire. The overwhelming answer to this question is that the fundamental reading problem for most dyslexic, or reading disabled, children involves difficulties acquiring accurate and fluent word identification skills (Morrison 1987; Stanovich 1988). In particular, most reading disabled children have great difficulty learning to acquire phonetically based reading strategies; they have difficulties learning letter sound correspondences, and, especially, they have difficulty applying these correspondences in "sounding out" words (Rack, Snowling, and Olson 1992). Children with reading disabilities are often unable to attain alphabetic or phonological reading skills fully. Not only does this limit their early independence in reading, but it probably also interferes with subsequent development of orthographic, or sight word reading strategies that are the basis for fluent reading (Share and Stanovich 1995).

Word Reading Processes in Skilled Readers

In order to understand why these early difficulties in acquiring phonetic reading skills interfere so strongly with normal reading growth in dyslexic children, we need to understand two important facts about skilled reading that were not clearly understood until recently. The first fact is that skilled readers, both children and adults, fixate almost every word in text as they read (Raynor and Pollatsek 1989). Skilled readers are able to process text rapidly, not because they selectively sample words and letters as they construct its meaning, but because they read the individual words so rapidly and with so little effort. Skilled readers process words as *orthographic units* (Ehri in press).

A key piece of knowledge here, and our second important fact about text processing in skilled readers, is that sight word representations (researchers call these orthographic representations because they represent the letter patterns in words) include information about all, or almost all, the letters in words. (For reviews, see Just and Carpenter 1987 and Patterson and Coltheart 1987.) Because many words are differentiated from one another by only one or two letters, a global, or gestalt image of a word is not sufficient to help recognize it reliably. Instead, the memory image used in reading words by sight must include information about all, or almost all the letters in a word's spelling. Even when reading very rapidly, the good reader extracts information about all the letters in a word as part of the recognition process.

To help the reader of this chapter understand the level of specificity of the representations skilled readers use when recognizing words, consider the following list of pairs of words: smoak-smoke, circus-sircus, wagon-wagun, ferst-first, trade-train, laugh-laff. It is not difficult for skilled readers to recognize instantly which word of each pair is the real word because the orthographic representation for each of these words in long-term memory contains information about all its letters. Marilyn Adams, in her book *Beginning to Read: Thinking and Learning about Print* (1990), summarizes these facts about word recognition processes in skilled readers this way:

> The most salient characteristic of skillful readers is the speed and effortlessness with which they seem able to breeze through text. Over time, many hypotheses have been offered to explain this remarkable facility: Do skillful readers recognize words as wholes, relying on their overall patterns or shapes rather than any closer analysis of their spellings? Do they use context to anticipate the wording of the text, such that they can confine visual analysis to its most important or least predictable words? Do they use context to anticipate the meanings of the words they will see, such that their comprehension consists as much of confirmation as of interpretation? As appealing as each of these hypotheses may have been, none is correct. It turns out instead, that skillful readers visually process virtually every individual letter of every word as they read, and this is true whether they are reading isolated words or meaningful text. (p. 409)

If the key to becoming a skilled reader is to acquire a large vocabulary of words that can be recognized fluently by sight, then the next question we must consider is how do good readers acquire these orthographic representations?

Processes Involved in the Normal Growth of Word Reading Skill

Share and his colleagues (Share 1995; Share and Jorm 1987; Share and Stanovich 1995) have recently presented a compelling case for the role of phonological reading skills as a critical base for the development of fully specified orthographic representations of words. In this model, emergent skills in phonological decoding provide the basis for acquiring accurate orthographic representations of words from the very beginning of the learning process. A central tenet of their argument is that if children use partial or complete phonological cues to derive an approximate pronunciation for a word in text, and combine this approximate pronunciation with contextual constraints to identify the fully correct pronunciation, the prior attention to individual letters involved in alphabetic decoding provides a solid basis for acquisition or refinement of an orthographic representation for the word. As children's increasingly developed alphabetic reading skills lead to more detailed analyses of the internal structure of words in print, they begin to acquire increasingly explicit and more fully specified orthographic representations.

It is important to note here that children encounter far too many new words in the later stages of elementary school for them all to be directly taught by teachers. For example, Nagy and Herman (1987) report analyses suggesting that the average fifth grader learns to read about 10,000 new words during the year! In order to be added to a child's vocabulary of sight words, a word must be encountered and pronounced correctly several times. Unless a child has the phonetic skills to insure that word reading is relatively accurate (guessing from context alone produces too many errors [Gough 1983]), it is extremely difficult to acquire enough accurate whole word representations to support fluent and accurate reading (Ehri in press).

To summarize, although skilled reading in older children depends very little on phonetic reading skills because most words are recognized "by sight," phonetic reading skills are critical in helping to acquire good sight vocabularies which are the basis of fluent word reading in text.

The Primary Cause of Dyslexic Children's Difficulties in Acquiring Accurate Word Reading Skill

If children with reading disabilities experience a bottleneck in their reading growth because of difficulties acquiring phonetic reading skills, what do we know about the causes of these difficulties? We have learned a great deal about this question in recent years, and there is now a strong consensus that the reading difficulties of most dyslexic children involve a dysfunction "in the phonological component of their natural capacity for language" (Liberman, Shankweiler, and Liberman 1989, p. 1). This dysfunction is expressed in performance limitations on a variety of nonreading tasks, such as those that assess sensitivity to the phonological structure of words, those that assess speed of access to phonological information in long-term memory, and those that examine short-term memory for verbal information (Shankweiler and Liberman 1989; Wagner and Torgesen 1987; Torgesen 1995). These intrinsic limitations in ability to process phonological information not only interfere with dyslexic children's understanding of how letters represent the sounds in words, but also limit the efficiency with which they can apply whatever understanding they are able to attain. Although there may be more than one subtype of specific developmental dyslexia (Castles and Coltheart 1993), the best described and most common subtype is phonologically based reading disability.

Of all the areas of phonological disability identified in children with dyslexia, the one that has been studied the most intensively is phonological awareness. *Phonological awareness* involves a more or less explicit understanding that words can be divided into segments of sound smaller than a syllable, as well as knowledge, or awareness, of the identity of individual phonemes themselves. A *phoneme* is the smallest unit of sound in a word that makes a difference in its meaning. For example, the word "cat" has three phonemes, /k/, /a/, /t/. It is different from the word "bat" in its first phoneme, different from the word "cut" in its second phoneme, and different from the word "cab" in its final phoneme. Phonemes usually correspond to single letters in print, except for cases like the word "that," in which the first phoneme is represented by two letters, or "which," in which the first and last phonemes are each represented by two letters. Then there is the oddball case of the letter "x" that represents two phonemes, /k/ and /s/, so that the word "ox" has three phonemes, and the word "exit" has five.

Phonological awareness emerges in young children as an initial sensitivity to the phonological structure of words, as is shown in the ability to notice rhyme, or to generate rhyming words. Children in kindergarten may also begin to notice that words can share beginning or ending sounds in common, particularly if this structure is pointed out by their teachers or parents. As children begin to learn about letters, letter names, and letter sounds, they acquire more explicit awareness of the phonemic structure of words, so that they can begin explicitly to segment words into their phonemes, or they can blend separately presented phonemes into sounds.

It should be pointed out here that initially at least, phonological awareness is not the same thing as "phonics." The word *phonics* is used to refer to reading skills involving the use of letter-sound correspondences to "sound out" words. Phonological awareness, on the other hand, is an oral language skill involving sensitivity to the phonological structure of spoken words. Tests of phonological awareness do not involve letters, but rather ask children to perform such tasks as categorizing words on the basis of similar beginning or ending sounds, deleting sounds from words to make other words (i.e., "What word do you have if you say 'card' without saying the /d/ sound?"; and blending sounds together to produce words (i.e., "If you blend these sounds together, /k/-/a/-/t/, what word do they make?") One of the most solidly established facts about early reading growth is that children who perform relatively poorly on tasks like these are highly likely to experience difficulties learning to read (Stanovich, Cunningham, and Cramer 1984; Torgesen, Wagner, and Rashotte 1994; Wagner, Torgesen, and Rashotte 1994). This level of awareness of the sounds in words is not required for speaking and listening because of our natural biological capacity for speech (Liberman, Shankweiler, and Liberman 1989), but it is required to understand the way that oral language is represented in written form.

Instructional Implications of Present Knowledge About Reading and Reading Disabilities

If the goal of preventive and remedial instruction for children with reading disabilities is to help them acquire reading skills similar to those of their non-disabled peers, then there are several very clear implications for instructional practice of current knowledge about skilled reading, reading acquisition processes, and reading disabilities. The content of reading instruction should seek to:

1. *Stimulate the growth of phonological awareness as the basis for understanding and applying the alphabetic principle in decoding novel words.* This principle is based on evidence that individual differences in phonological awareness are causally related to the acquisition of effective word reading skills.

2. *Foster the early growth of alphabetic reading skills as the basis for early independence in word identification and gradual development of fully specified orthographic representations.* This principle is based on knowledge that the path to accurate and fluent visually based word reading ability goes through the early development and utilization of phonetic reading strategies. This may be our most controversial principle because this involves teaching to the weakness of dyslexic children rather than to their *strengths*. Previous research has also shown that it is very difficult for

many dyslexic children to acquire functional phonetic reading skills (Lovett et al. 1990; Lyon 1985; Snowling and Hulme 1989). Nevertheless, given the importance of phonetic reading skills in most scientific accounts of reading growth (Adams 1990; Share and Stanovich 1995; Vellutino 1991), it seems essential to address this issue if dyslexic children are to become functional, adaptive, and independent readers.

3. *Build accurate and fluent print based, visually driven, word identification skills.* This principle requires that instruction address the question of helping dyslexic children utilize their phonetic reading skills and other word identification strategies to build a rich orthographic reading vocabulary. For example, we know that phonological reading skills provide necessary, but not entirely sufficient, support for the development of good orthographic reading ability. That is, a child may be able to identify words accurately by using phonological/analytic strategies, but if these skills are not applied in extensive exposure to print, the development of a rich orthographic reading vocabulary will not take place (Cunningham and Stanovich 1991; Stanovich and West 1989).

4. *Assist dyslexic children to apply their fluent and accurate word reading skills to comprehend the meaning of print.* Although children whose general verbal abilities are adequately developed already posses most of the knowledge and skill required to construct the meaning of print, they still may need some special help to enhance their reading comprehension. For example, if the acquisition of their word reading skills has been slow, and most of their reading instruction has focused on word identification skills, they may lag behind their normally developing peers in understanding and utilizing a range of reading strategies that can enhance print comprehension, or repair it if it breaks down (Brown, Palincsar, and Purcell 1986).

In addition to these general guidelines for the content of reading instruction, at least three aspects of the methodology of instruction can be derived from current knowledge of the difficulties that dyslexic children face in learning to read. For children with specific developmental reading disabilities:

1. *Instruction must be more explicit and comprehensive.* Most of the knowledge that is acquired in the process of *normal* reading development is discovered during interactions with print. As children read, they notice useful generalizations about print-sound relationships, and they acquire a great deal of word specific

knowledge as well (the orthographic representations that are required for fluent reading). Because of their weaknesses in the area of phonological processing, children with reading disabilities require explicit and systematic instruction to help them acquire the knowledge and strategies necessary for decoding print. As Gaskins et al. (1997) have pointed out, "First graders who are at risk for failure in learning to read do not discover what teachers leave unsaid about the complexities of word learning. As a result, it is important to teach them procedures for learning words" (p. 325).

2. *Instruction must be more intensive.* Increased explicitness requires that more things be taught directly which implies that reading disabled children will need to be provided with either more instructional time or a much smaller teacher-pupil ratio if they are to learn reading skills at close to normal rates. Another factor that underlines the need for more intensive instruction is the fact that children with phonological disabilities learn critical decoding skills more slowly than other children and will require more repetition in order to establish critical decoding skills.

3. *Instruction must be more supportive, both emotionally and cognitively.* The needs of children with reading disabilities for more positive emotional support in the form of encouragement, feedback, and positive reinforcement is widely understood. However, their potential need for more cognitive support, in the form of carefully "scaffolded" instruction, is less widely appreciated. Scaffolded instruction involves finely tuned interactions between teacher and child that support the child in accomplishing a task that he/she could not do without the teacher's help (Stone 1989). This type of teacher-student dialogue directly shows the child what kind of processing, or thinking, needs to be done in order to complete the task successfully. In general, a scaffolded interaction consists of four elements: (a) the student is presented with a task such as reading or spelling a word (i.e., tries to spell the word "fled"); (b) the student makes a response that is incorrect in some way, or indicates that he or she does not know how to proceed (i.e., spells it "fed"); (c) the teacher asks a question that focuses the child's attention on a first step in the solution process, or that draws attention to a required piece of information ("You're right that the word does start with the /f/ sound, and when you say fled, what do you hear coming right after the /f/?"); (d) another response from the child ("I hear the /l/ sound"). This kind of interaction between teacher and child would continue until the child had been led to accomplish the

task successfully. The point of this type of instructional interaction is that the child is led to discover the information or strategies that are critical to accomplishing the task, rather than simply being told what to do. As Juel has recently described (1996), the ability to offer scaffolded support while children are acquiring reading skills may have increasing importance as the severity of the child's disability increases.

PREVENTIVE AND REMEDIAL INTERVENTIONS FOR CHILDREN WITH PHONOLOGICALLY BASED READING DISABILITIES

In the remainder of this paper, I will briefly discuss two intervention studies that we have been involved with for the past three years. My colleagues on these studies include Richard Wagner, Carol Rashotte, Ann Alexander, Kyjta Voeller, and Tim Conway. Both of these studies involve relatively intense interventions, as one of our goals was to determine the extent to which reading skills can be "normalized" in children with severe phonologically based reading disabilities. One of the studies takes a preventive approach, while the other examines remedial procedures.

A Prevention Study Involving Relatively Long-term Instruction

Children were selected for participation in this study in the first semester of kindergarten based on their test scores of letter name knowledge and on a measure of phonological awareness demonstrated to identify children at risk for early reading difficulties (Torgesen and Burgess in press). Statistical procedures were used to identify children likely to be in the bottom 10% of readers by second grade. Children who obtained an estimated verbal IQ below 75 were excluded from the study.

The 180 children in the final sample were randomly assigned to four instructional conditions: (1) phonological awareness training at an oral/motor level plus synthetic phonics instruction (PASP); (2) implicit phonological awareness training plus phonics instructions embedded within real word reading and spelling activities (EP); (3) a regular classroom support group receiving individual instruction to support the goals of the regular classroom reading program (RCS); and, (4) a no-treatment control group. The RCS group received individual tutoring in the activities and skills taught in the regular classroom reading program. Although this condition did not involve an experimental curriculum per se, a potential advantage of this group over the other two was that its instructional activities were closely co-ordinated with the instructional activities taking place in the child's regular classroom. It was also included as a control against the possibility that the effectiveness of the experimental curricula was primarily the result of intensity (one-to-one) of instruction rather than content or method.

Children in each instructional condition were provided with 80 minutes of one-to-one supplemental instruction in reading each week during the 2½ year intervention period. Two of these 20 minute instructional sessions were led by certified teachers, and two of the sessions were led by instructional aides who followed the teacher's instructions to reinforce what the children learned in the previous teacher-led session. Over the course of the study, the children received a total of about 88 hours of supplemental instruction (47 hours from teachers and 41 hours from aides).

The primary instructional contrast between the two experimental/instructional conditions (PASP and EP) involved the degree of explicitness of instruction in phonological awareness and alphabetic reading skills as well as the extent of focused practice on these skills. The most alphabetically explicit approach, which we have labeled Phonological Awareness Plus Synthetic Phonics (PASP) was based almost exclusively on the *Auditory Discrimination in Depth* method developed by Patricia and Charles Lindamood (1984).

In this program, phonological awareness is stimulated by helping children discover the articulatory positions and mouth movements associated with the different phonemes in the English language. As part of this instruction, the children also learn labels for each phoneme that are descriptive of these mouth movements and positions (i.e., "lip popper," "tip tapper," "scraper"). Once the children attain a high criterion of knowledge in oral awareness they engage in an extensive series of problem solving exercises that involve presenting sequences of phonemes with either mouth-form pictures or colored blocks. This training focuses on helping them acquire sensitivity to the sequences of sounds in syllables, and it also enables them to learn to represent these sequences with concrete visual objects.

Throughout the program, instructional interactions consist primarily of questions that the teacher asks in order to help the child "discover" that he or she can "think about" the sounds in words by both feeling what happens in the mouth and hearing the sounds with the ear. The object of this scaffolded instruction is to help the children learn to verify the nature and order of the phonemes in words from their own sensory experience. As they learn to label each phoneme with a descriptive name, they are also associating specific letters with each phoneme. So, once they become facile at representing sequences of sounds with concrete objects, it becomes natural to represent them with letters.

The PASP program provided extensive practice in decoding (reading) and encoding (spelling) individual words that followed regular patterns, but children were also introduced to the idea that some words "don't play fair," so that parts of them simply have to be learned by sight. As soon as the children learned to decode words using a small number of consonants and vowels, they began reading small books using a vocabulary that was "protected" phonologically. Whenever the children read in books, the teachers emphasized both accurate decoding and self-correction of errors as well as comprehending and enjoying the stories that were read. As soon as children began work on multi-syllabic words, they read orally from "trade books" or books they brought from class. During oral reading activities, they were encouraged to rely on their skills in phonological decoding, but were also encouraged to ask whether the pronunciation of an unfamiliar word "made sense" in the context of the story. During second grade, the children also received direct, fluency guiding practice in recognizing words from a list of words that occurred with high frequency in printed English.

The other instructional approach, which we labeled Embedded Phonics (EP), provided less intensive, but still systematic, phonics training in the context of early and meaningful experiences in reading and writing text. In its early phases, the instructional periods in this program consisted of four main activities: (1) learning to recognize small groups of whole words by using word level drill and word games, (2) instruction in letter-sound correspondences in the context of sight words being learned, (3) writing the words in sentences, and (4) reading the sentences that were written. Some letter sounds (short vowel, r-controlled vowels) were taught through memorization of picture-word cards, but most grapheme-phoneme correspondences were taught in the context of writing activities. The children also received direct instruction in a small number of highly useful phonics generalizations. Stimulation of phonological awareness was accomplished during writing activities in which the children were asked to identify the beginning and subsequent sounds in words before writing them. For many beginning words, they were also asked to check their spellings to see if they represented all the sounds in the words.

The words the children learned were taken from a basal series that contained stories. The stories were read orally after the words in them were learned, and the primary emphasis during the entire "basal" phase was on acquiring word level reading skills (sight vocabulary and supportive alphabetic decoding skills). After the children finished the first grade reader in the basal series, the emphasis of the program shifted from learning to read by writing to learning to read by reading. Less time was spent on individual word drills and more time was spent on reading stories from the basal series as well as trade books. Teacher-student dialogues during reading focused heavily on constructing the meaning of the stories that were read, although continual support for accurate decoding and self-correction were also provided during text reading. Children were explicitly taught to integrate phonological decoding skills with use of context to help determine the identity of unknown words in the text.

Preliminary Results of our Prevention Study

The ultimate effectiveness of the interventions provided in this study can only be determined by long-term follow-up of the children as they move through elementary school and into middle and high school. The most important test of any preventive measure is how effectively it establishes a foundation of reading skills that can be used to sustain continued growth in reading after the intervention ceases. At this point, we have data available from the final testing at the end of the intervention period, and they indicate that children in one of our intervention groups may have established a significantly stronger foundation in basic reading skills than children in the other groups.

Performance of the children at the end of second grade on several of our outcome measures is provided in table I. The data in this table represent the performance of all children who remained in the study at the end of the instructional period. Most of the children were finishing second grade, although a total of about 26% of the children from the total sample were retained in either kindergarten or first grade, and so were finishing first grade. Rates of retention differed across instructional conditions, with children in the PASP (Phonological Awareness Plus Synthetic Phonics) group showing the smallest rate (9%), and rates for the EP (Embedded Phonics), RCS (Regular Classroom Reading Program), and no treatment group being 25%, 30%, and 41%, respectively. In this chapter, we present results for first and second grade children grouped together because we are interested in showing the overall effect of each type of intervention.

In table I, scores on the Word Attack and Word Identification tests are presented in age based standard score units so that we can estimate the extent to which the reading skills of children in each group approached normal levels for children their age. Notice, for example, that children in the PASP group attained a standard score of 99.4 on

Table I. Reading, Phonological Awareness, and Spelling Scores for All Groups at the End of Second Grade

Measure	Group							
	Control (n = 32)		RCS (n = 37)		PASP (n = 33)		EP (n = 36)	
	X	SD	X	SD	X	SD	X	SD
Blend Phonemes[1]	16.3	5.4	16.8	5.2	18.0	4.9	17.4	3.6
Phoneme Elision[2]	13.0	4.9	12.0	4.9	15.8	5.7*	11.9	4.5
Phoneme Segmentation[3]	7.1	3.2	7.3	3.3	9.2	3.8*	7.3	2.8
Word Attack[4]	81.6	17.1	86.7	19.4	99.4	16.8*	86.7	13.1
Word Identification[5]	86.3	17.8	92.0	15.5	98.2	17.9	92.1	14.5
Passage Comp.[6]	85.2	15.7	86.4	14.8	91.7	14.5	87.4	15.6
Word Efficiency[7]	16.6	15.2	29.4	16.6	36.4	17.1	30.8	15.7
Nonword Efficiency[8]	10.0	8.8	11.2	12.1	20.5	13.8*	11.7	9.7
Developmental Spell[9]	22.6	4.3	22.5	5.2	25.5	3.7*	22.6	5.6

Note – on all comparisons marked with an asterisk, the overall comparison among groups was statistically significant, and the PASP group obtained significantly higher scores than children in the other groups.

[1]*Blending Phonemes Test*—a measure of phonological awareness that requires children to recognize words from separately presented phonemes (i.e., /k/-/a/-/t/ = cat)

[2]*Phoneme Elision*—a measure of phonological awareness that requires children to form a new word by deleting a specific sound from a target word (i.e., delete /d/ from card = car)

[3]*Phoneme Segmentation*—a measure of phonological awareness that requires children to pronounce the phonemes in words separately (i.e., cat = /k/-/a/-/t/)

[4]*Word Attack* subtest from the *Woodcock Reading Mastery Test-Revised* (Woodcock 1989)

[5]*Word Identification* subtest from the *Woodcock Reading Mastery Test-Revised.*

[6]*Passage Comprehension* subtest from the *Woodcock Reading Mastery Test-revised.*

[7]*Word Reading Efficiency*—a measure of fluency in word reading that requires one to read as many words as possible in 45 seconds from a word list that gradually increases in difficulty

[8]*Nonword Reading Efficiency*—a measure of fluency in alphabetic reading that requires children to read as many nonwords as possible in 45 seconds from a list that increases from two phoneme nonwords to 10 phoneme words.

[9]*Developmental Spelling Test*—children were asked to spell the words *lap, sick, pretty, train,* and *elephant.* Responses were scored to indicate the phonological accuracy of the spelling.

the Word Attack subtest and a score of 98.2 on the Word Identification measure. These scores are right at average levels for children their age. We were also able to estimate an age based standard score for Word and Nonword Reading Efficiency measure because of extensive use of these measures with random samples of children of the same age in our local school district. For the Nonword efficiency measure, the average standard score of children in the PASP group were the same as "average" children in terms of both accuracy and fluency. Table I also indicates that the PASP group had a significant performance advantage on several measures of phonological awareness, and on a measure (Developmental Spelling) that assessed children's use of phonetic strategies in spelling. Overall differences on the Word Identification subtest just failed to reach the required level of statistical reliability. Table I also shows that the superior alphabetic reading skills of children in the PASP group have not yet produced significant differences among groups in a standardized measure of reading comprehension. However, it should be noted that the comprehension standard score for children in the PASP condition was almost exactly equivalent to the average verbal IQ (91 for the group). It is likely that this comprehension score is limited by the children's general language comprehension ability and does not reflect the influence of poor word reading skills, as is commonly the case with children who have phonological reading disabilities.

Although the alphabetic reading skills of children in the PASP condition approached average levels for the group as a whole, there was considerable variability in response to instruction within the group. Within this condition, 24% of the children remained more than one standard deviation below normal in these skills at the end of training. This means that the PASP treatment, as delivered in this study, was relatively ineffective in "normalizing" the alphabetic reading skills of approximately 2.4% of children in the total population from which our treatment sample (bottom 10%) was selected.

The four children with the weakest alphabetic reading skills in the PASP group obtained standard scores of 63, 73, 74, and 78, and the standard scores of these same children on the Word Identification subtest were 81, 69, 74, and 85, respectively. Clearly, these children could be said to have continuing reading disabilities in spite of the $2^1/2$ years of preventive intervention they received.

Our Remedial Study with 8- to 11-year-old Children

The children participating in this study had already been identified by the public school system as learning disabled. Children were initially nominated by their teachers as those having the greatest difficulties acquiring word level reading skills, and then we verified their difficulties in alphabetic reading and phonological awareness through a series of tests of our own.

One of the most unusual things about this study was the intensity of the instruction provided to the children. Students were seen individually in two hour sessions, five days a week, for about eight weeks, a total of 80 hours of instruction. Following the intensive instruction, students were seen in their learning disabilities classroom by the project teacher for one hour a week for eight weeks. The purpose of this follow-up instruction was to help the children apply their newly developed reading skills to the kinds of assignments they receive in the classroom.

The *Auditory Discrimination In–Depth Program* was used in essentially the same way as the prevention study, with all children starting at the beginning of the program and randomly assigned to the same two experimental/instructional conditions. The overall instructional philosophy and balance of activities for the embedded phonics curriculum was the same, but instruction was designed specifically to fill in the "gaps" of each child's alphabetic and word level reading skills rather than teach a systematic curriculum from the beginning. The teachers in this study were always more highly trained and experienced than those participating in the prevention study.

Training has now been completed for 51 children with complete pre-, mid-, and post-test data available for 40 children. We also have one year follow-up data on a smaller group of 21 children. The large gains that children in both instructional conditions are making in the accuracy of their generalized alphabetic reading skills are the most

Table II. Reading Outcomes After 80 Hours of Individualized Tutorial Instruction

	Group							
	ADD (n = 21)				EP (n = 19)			
	pretest		posttest		pretest		posttest	
	X	SD	X	SD	X	SD	X	SD
Word Attack[1]	67.5	12.6	94.8	7.5	69.2	10.7	90.0	9.0
Word Identification[2]	68.4	9.0	82.4	12.1	65.7	9.6	82.7	9.3
Passage Comp.[3]	82.0	12.8	91.0	9.3	85.6	9.7	93.5	8.6
Nonword Efficiency[4]	72.4	10.1	83.2	12.3	78.9	11.6	85.8	12.1
Word Efficiency[5]	66.8	12.3	74.2	13.2	67.3	12.5	76.3	12.9

Note – This table contains scores for each test in standard score units (Mean = 100, SD =15.) The three subtests from the *Woodcock Reading Mastery Test-Revised* used norms based on a national sample. For the Word Efficiency and Nonword Efficiency test, local norms were used to derive standard scores.

[1]*Word Attack* subtest from the *Woodcock Reading Mastery Test-Revised* (Woodcock, 1989)

[2]*Word Identification* subtest from the *Woodcock Reading Mastery Test-Revised.*

[3]*Passage Comprehension* subtest from the *Woodcock Reading Mastery Test-Revised.*

[4]*Nonword Reading Efficiency*—a measure of fluency in alphabetic reading that requires children to read as many nonwords as possible in 45 seconds from a list that increases from two phoneme nonwords to 10 phoneme words.

[5]*Word Reading Efficiency*—a measure of fluency in word reading that requires one to read as many words as possible in 45 seconds from a word list that gradually increases in difficulty.

striking features of the results thus far. Table II presents pre- and posttest results for some of our basic reading measures. Children in both groups have moved from substantially below average in performance on measures of alphabetic reading up into the average range. This change represents from about one and a half to two years of growth in this skill over the 80 hours of instruction. Although differences between groups in average growth of alphabetic reading skills are not statistically reliable at this point, a higher proportion of children in the EP group (26%) compared with the ADD group (9%) remains substantially impaired (more than one standard deviation below average) in alphabetic reading accuracy at the end of the instruction period.

The children have also experienced substantial growth in their ability to recognize real words and to comprehend what they read, although these changes have not been so dramatic as those for alphabetic reading skills. In contrast to children in the prevention study, changes in *fluency* of basic word reading processes has lagged substantially behind changes in accuracy. The relative change in fluency of both nonword and real word reading is about half of what has been observed for improvements in accuracy.

Figure 1 presents data for the 21 children for whom one-year follow-up testing is now available. In this figure, the children's raw scores on the Word Attack and Word Identification subtests from the *Woodcock Reading Mastery Test-Revised* are plotted as a function of their age in months, with the assumed starting point for all children being the same at the beginning of school. The figure not only illustrates the dramatic alteration in growth occurring as a result of the intensive interventions used in this study, but it also shows continuing growth in average reading skills in the year following the intervention. The curved line at the top of these graphs represents normal growth for each skill in the national standardization sample.

Concluding Comments

I began this chapter by pointing out that recent advances in our understanding of reading and reading disabilities has established a useful context for more focused and interpretable intervention research than was possible in the past. One way that our new knowledge about reading disabilities is helpful is in the guidance it gives us in the selection of subjects. The consensus that phonological processing difficulties are the core problem in most cases of reading disability allows us to select more homogeneous and theoretically coherent samples of children to study. In addition, the information we have about skilled readers and the normal reading acquisition process allows us to focus on specific instructional goals.

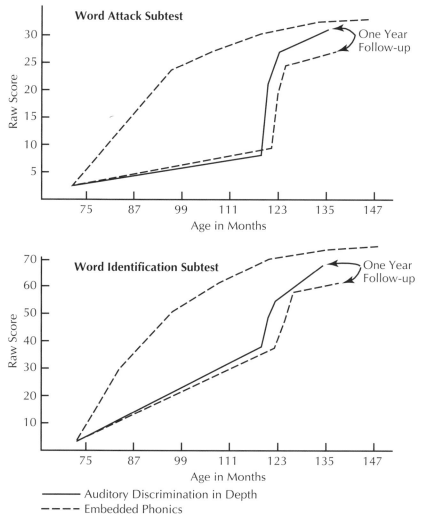

Figure 1.   Change in raw scores as a function of age for children receiving 80 hours of intensive intervention between the ages of eight and eleven.

From our studies, we know that it is clearly possible to teach children with phonologically based reading disabilities to employ alphabetic reading skills at levels approximating average performance, at least for accuracy. The results from our prevention study are consistent with an earlier preventive study reported by Rebecca Felton and colleagues (Brown and Felton 1990; Felton 1993) in that they show near average levels of performance on phonetic decoding tasks for the group as a whole. As in our study, the instructional approach that provided the most explicit instruction in the alphabetic code produced the most substantial growth in this skill.

Until we have adequate follow-up data on these children, we really will not be able to answer questions about the impact of stimulating alphabetic reading skills on subsequent growth in orthographic reading ability. At present, we do not have evidence from our prevention study that the group with the strongest alphabetic reading skills showed a correspondingly strong effect on a measure of sight word vocabulary. However, logically it should take some time for newly acquired alphabetic reading skills to have an impact on growth in sight word vocabulary, so our current tests of immediate training outcomes do not adequately answer this question.

A recently reported study by Olson et al. (in press) that reported one-year follow-up results did not find a differential effect on subsequent growth in sight word vocabulary between two groups who had different levels of alphabetic reading skills, resulting from differences in their instructional programs. Although the group with stronger alphabetic reading skills at the end of training retained their advantage in this area one year later, they did not show a faster rate of increase in their orthographic reading skills than the other group. Since this study used a relatively short training period, the authors suggested that, even though one of the groups was more accurate in phonetic reading, their skills may not yet have become sufficiently automatic or effortless for them to be used regularly while reading text. As we mentioned earlier, phonetic reading skills are probably a necessary but not sufficient cause of growth in sight word reading ability. They will not be helpful if they are not routinely applied when children are reading text.

There is ample evidence, both in our own data and in that of others (Wasik and Slavin 1993), that more intensive instruction in word level reading skills can improve reading comprehension in children with reading disabilities when compared to children not receiving special instruction. However, we still do not have solid research evidence that explicitly phonetic methods produce greater gains in comprehension than those emphasizing whole word, or context oriented instruction. This should not be taken as a contradiction to the recommended elements of instruction outlined earlier; rather, it merely reflects the relatively short-term, limited nature of the instructional research that has been conducted thus far.

All of the scientifically viable, well-controlled intervention research to date has involved relatively brief and highly focused interventions. The goal of the research has been to study the power of various methods to stimulate relatively short-term growth in specific, word level reading skills. Although this kind of research can provide guidance about the elements of effective instruction for the specific reading skills it targets, it frequently does not carry the instruction far enough to insure that the skills in question are developed to a point that they can function autonomously during complex text processing activities. As a case in point, phonetic reading skills must operate relatively fluently before children will rely on them as an aid to word identification while they are reading text. If these analytic skills remain slow and labored, even though they enhance reading accuracy, they may not be used because they make reading too difficult. Before we are able to answer fundamental questions about the conditions that must be in place for children with severe phonologically based reading disabilities to learn to read normally, we must find ways to conduct research that addresses all elements of the hierarchy of skills in reading within the same study. From numerous discussions with highly skilled reading clinicians, it is clear that many children will require far more than the 80 hours of one-to-one instruction we have been able to provide in our studies thus far. Although the body of knowledge we currently have about reading growth and reading disabilities provides strong guidance about the elements of effective instruction for children with phonologically based reading disabilities, we have yet to demonstrate what a "complete package" of necessary instructional elements, spread over what period of time, will be most effective in helping these children acquire normal reading skills.

The research reported in this chapter was supported by grant number HD23340 and HD30988 from the National Institute of Child Health and Human Development, and by grants from the National Center for Learning Disabilities, and the Donald D. Hammill Foundation

REFERENCES

Adams, M. J. 1990. *Beginning to Read: Thinking and Learning about Print.* Cambridge, MA: MIT Press.

Beck, I. L., and Juel, C. 1995. The role of decoding in learning to read. *American Educator* 19:8–20.

Beck, I. A., and McKeown, M. G. 1991. Conditions of vocabulary acquisition. In *Handbook of Reading Research*, Volume 2, eds. R. Barr, M. L. Kamil, P. Mosenthal, and P. D. Pearson. New York: Longman.

Brown, I. S., and Felton, R. H. 1990. Effects of instruction on beginning reading skills in children at risk for reading disability. *Reading and Writing: An Interdisciplinary Journal* 2:223–41.

Brown, A. L., Palincsar, A. S., and Purcell, L. 1986. Poor readers: Teach, don't label. In *The School Achievement of Minority Children: New Perspective*, ed. U. Neisser. Hillsdale, NJ: Lawrence Erlbaum Associates.

Castles, A., and Coltheart, M. 1993. Varieties of developmental dyslexia. *Cognition* 47: 149–80.

Clark, D. B. 1988. *Dyslexia: Theory and Practice of Remedial Instruction*. Parkton, MD: York Press.

Cunningham, A. E., and Stanovich, K. E. 1991. Tracking the unique effects of print exposure in children: Association with vocabulary, general knowledge, and spelling. *Journal of Educational Psychology* 83:264–74.

Ehri, L. C. in press. Grapheme-phoneme knowledge is essential for learning to read words in English. In *Word Recognition in Beginning Reading*, eds. J. Metsala and L. Ehri. Hillsdale, NJ: Lawrence Erlbaum Associates.

Felton, R. H. 1993. Effects of instruction on the decoding skills of children with phonological-processing problems. *Journal of Learning Disabilities* 26:583–89.

Gaskins, I. W., Ehri, L. C., Cress, C., O'Hara, C., and Donnelly, K. 1997. Procedures for word learning: Making discoveries about words. *The Reading Teacher* 50:312–27.

Gough, P. B. 1996. How children learn to read and why they fail. *Annals of Dyslexia* 46:3–20.

Gough, P. B. 1983. Context, form and interaction. In *Eye Movements in Reading*, ed. K. Raynor. New York: Academic Press.

Gough, P. B., and Hillinger, M. L. 1980. Learning to read: An unnatural act. *Bulletin of The Orton Society* 30:171–76.

Hoover, W. A., and Gough, P. B. 1990. The simple view of reading. *Reading and Writing* 2:127–60.

Juel, C. 1996. What makes literacy tutoring effective? *Reading Research Quarterly* 31:268–89.

Just, M. A., and Carpenter, P. A. 1987. *The Psychology of Reading and Language Comprehension*. Boston: Allyn & Bacon.

Liberman, I. Y., Shankweiler, D., and Liberman, A. M. 1989. The alphabetic principle and learning to read. In *Phonology and Reading Disability: Solving the Reading Puzzle*, eds. D. Shankweiler and I. Y. Liberman. Ann Arbor, MI: University of Michigan Press.

Lindamood, C. H., and Lindamood, P. C. 1984. *Auditory Discrimination in Depth*. Austin, TX: PRO-ED, Inc.

Lovett, M. W., Warren-Chaplin, P. M., Ransby, M. J., and Borden, S. L. 1990. Training the word recognition skills of reading disabled children: Treatment and transfer effects. *Journal of Educational Psychology* 82:769–80.

Lyon, G. R. 1985. Identification and remediation of learning disability subtypes: Preliminary findings. *Learning Disabilities Focus* 1:21–35.

Morrison, F. J. 1987. The nature of reading disability: Toward an integrative framework. In *Handbook of Cognitive, Social, and Neuropsychological Aspects of Learning Disabilities*, ed. S. Ceci. Hillsdale, NJ: Lawrence Erlbaum Associates.

Nagy, W. E., and Herman, P. A. 1987. Breadth and depth of vocabulary knowledge: Implications for acquisition and instruction. In *The Nature of Vocabulary Acquisition*, eds. M. McKeown and M. Curtis. Hillsdale, NJ: Lawrence Erlbaum Associates.

Olson, R. K., Wise, B., Johnson, M., and Ring, J. in press. The etiology and remediation of phonologically based word recognition and spelling disabilities: Are phonological deficits the "hole" story? In *Foundations of Reading Acquisition*, ed. B. Blachman. Mahway, NJ: Lawrence Erlbaum Associates.

Palincsar, A. S., and Brown, A. L. 1984. Reciprocal teaching of comprehension-fostering and comprehension-monitoring activities. *Cognition and Instruction* 1:117–75.

Patterson, K. E., and Coltheart, V. 1987. Phonological processing in reading: A tutorial review. In *Attention and Performance*, Vol 12: The Psychology of Reading, ed. M. Coltheart. Hillsdale, NJ: Lawrence Erlbaum Associates.

Rack, J. P., Snowling, M. J., and Olson, R. K. 1992. The nonword reading deficit in developmental dyslexia: A review. *Reading Research Quarterly* 27:29–53.

Rayner, K., and Pollatsek, A. 1989. *The Psychology of Reading*. Englewood Cliffs, NJ: Prentice Hall.

Shankweiler, D., and Liberman, I. Y. 1989. *Phonology and Reading Disability*. Ann Arbor, MI: University of Michigan Press.

Share, D. L. 1995. Phonological recoding and self-teaching: Sine qua non or reading acquisition. *Cognition* 55:151–218.

Share, D. L., and Jorm, A. F. 1987. Segmental analysis: Co-requisite to reading, vital for self-teaching, requiring phonological memory. *European Bulletin of Cognitive Psychology* 7:5019–13.

Share, D. L., and Stanovich, K. E. 1995. Cognitive processes in early reading development: A model of acquisition and individual differences. *Issues in Education: Contributions from Educational Psychology* 1:1–57.

Snowling, M., and Hulme, C. 1989. A longitudinal case study of developmental phonological dyslexia. *Cognitive neuropsychology* 6:379–401.

Stanovich, K. E. 1988. Explaining the differences between the dyslexic and the garden-variety poor reader: The phonological-core variable-difference model. *Journal of Learning Disabilities* 21:590–604.

Stanovich, K. E., Cunningham, A. E., and Cramer, B. B. 1984. Assessing phonological awareness in kindergarten children: Issues of task comparability. *Journal of Experimental Child Psychology* 38:175–90.

Stanovich, K. E., and West, R. F. 1989. Exposure to print and orthographic processing. *Reading Research Quarterly* 24:402–33.

Stone, A. 1989. Improving the effectiveness of strategy training for learning disabled students: The role of communicational dynamics. *Remedial and Special Education* 10:35–41.

Torgesen, J. K., and Burgess, S. R. in press. Consistency of reading-related phonological processes throughout early childhood: Evidence from longitudinal correlational and instructional studies. In *Word Recognition in Beginning Literacy*, eds. J. Metsala and L. Ehri. Mahway, NJ: Lawrence Erlbaum Associates, Inc.

Torgesen, J. K. 1995. A model of memory from an information processing perspective: The special case of phonological memory. In *Attention, Memory, and Executive Function: Issues in Conceptualization and Measurement*, ed. G. Reid Lyon. Baltimore, MD: Brookes Publishing Co.

Torgesen, J. K., Wagner, R. K., and Rashotte, C. A. 1994. Longitudinal studies of phonological processing and reading. *Journal of Learning Disabilities* 27:276–86.

Vellutino, F. R. 1991. Introduction to three studies on reading acquisition: Convergent findings on theoretical foundations of code-oriented versus whole-language approaches to reading instruction. *Journal of Educational Psychology* 83:437–44.

Wagner, R. K., and Torgesen, J. K. 1987. The nature of phonological processing and its causal role in the acquisition of reading skills. *Psychological Bulletin* 101:192–212.

Wagner, R. K., Torgesen, J. K., and Rashotte, C. A. 1994. The development of reading-related phonological processing abilities: New evidence of bi-directional causality from a latent variable longitudinal study. *Developmental Psychology* 30:73–87.

Wasik, B. A., and Slavin, R. E. 1993. Preventing early reading failure with one-to-one tutoring: A review of five programs. *Reading Research Quarterly* 28:179–98.

Section • V

Outcomes and Predictions

Chapter • 11

The Long-term Prognosis of Learning Disabled Children
A Review of Studies (1954–1993)

Paul Satz,
Stephen Buka,
Lewis Lipsitt, and
Larry Seidman

In the past decade, enormous strides have been made in understanding the nature of specific reading disabilities, which comprise roughly 80% of the learning disabled (LD) population (Norman and Zigmond 1980). These developments have included sharper definitional criteria and prevalence estimates (Fletcher et al. 1992; Shaywitz, Fletcher, and Shaywitz 1995); identification of putative neural and brain metabolic substrates primarily in the left cerebral hemisphere and planum temporale (Larsen 1990; Hynd et al. 1990; Larsen, Hoien, and Odegaard 1992); identification of a phonological processing deficit as the core defect in most children and adults with reading, spelling, and writing disorders (Pennington 1991); and evidence that genetic factors are linked to family history of reading disorders as well as to the phonological code (Pennington et al. 1987; Pennington and Smith 1988). Despite these advances, and the inevitable controversies that they engender, one major domain of inquiry continues to remain unclear—namely, the long-term outcome of reading disabled and learning disabled children.

In the past 25 years there have been five reviews on the prognosis of these children over time (Herjanic and Penick 1972; Watson, Watson, and Fredd 1982; Schonhaut and Satz 1983; Kavale 1988; Spreen 1988). While most of these reviews have reported persistence of reading, spelling, and writing problems at various follow-up periods for a majority of childhood cases, the conclusions have been tempered by the different number of studies reported in each review and differences in methodology and results across studies. In order to address these problems, recent reviews (Schonhaut and Satz 1983; Kavale 1988; Spreen 1988) have focused primarily on reading and learning problems which, in recent years, have been shown to have different cognitive and underlying brain substrate than attention deficit hyperactivity disorders (ADHD). Although overlap in symptoms has long been reported between these disorders, the association has generally been small when more rigorous definitional criteria have been employed (Pennington 1991). These efforts have led recently to lower co-morbidity estimates and, consequently, lower potential threats to syndromal validity.

SCHONHAUT AND SATZ (1983) REVIEW

This review will be discussed briefly because it provides a conceptual framework—to be used in this updated review chapter—for evaluating and classifying studies based on key methodological criteria. Twenty-one studies (1959–1978) were identified that were shown to vary markedly in terms of sample selection and size, outcome measures, comparison groups, follow-up intervals, and results. Three studies omitted in the 1983 review (Herman 1959; Bell and Aftanas 1972; Frauenheim 1978), have now been incorporated in this review. The studies were evaluated in three ways. The first approach employed a box-score count of outcome results (good, mixed, poor) for all studies, independent of scientific merit. The second approach involved a series of box-score counts for studies selected for merit on one of five important methodological criteria noted above (e.g., sample selection, follow up). The third approach entailed a critique of only those studies selected for merit, based on a composite scale derived from the preceding methodological criteria. For purposes of brevity, only the general box-score outcomes (Approach 1) and methodologically stronger studies (Approach 3) will be discussed for the original Schonhaut and Satz (1983) review.

The general outcome results can be seen in table I. Without weighing scientific merit, they revealed four good outcomes, fifteen poor outcomes, and two mixed. While results showed almost four

Table I.   LD Outcomes: Early Studies (*n* = 21) Schonhaut and Satz Review (1983)

Good (G)	Mixed (M)	Poor (P)
Robinson et al. (1962)	Silver et al. (1965)	*Herman (1954)
Balow et al. (1965)	Kline (!975)	Carter (1964)
Preston et al. (1967)	*Bell et al. (1972)	Howden (1967)
Rawson (1968)		Hardy (1968)
		Dykman et al. (1973)
		Muehl et al. (1973)
		Gottesman et al. (1975)
		Rutter et al. (1976)
		Trites et al. (1976)
		Rourke et al. (1977)
		Ackerman et al. (1977)
		*Frauenheim (1978)
		Satz et al. (1978)
		Spreen (1978)

Box-Score Outcomes: 4(G), 3(M), 14(P).
*Not included in original review.

times as many poor outcomes, these findings could be misleading if the methodology of studies finding good outcomes was better than those finding poor outcomes. For this reason, it is important to identify a set of minimally sufficient criteria to be employed in a follow-up study of learning disabled children.

Schonhaut and Satz (1983) identified five criteria considered necessary, if not sufficient, to determine the prognosis of LD children: (1) an adequate follow-up period, (2) a sufficiently large sample size (at baseline and follow up), (3) a satisfactory method of sample selection, (4) an adequate comparison group, and (5) a valid and objective measure of reading/learning ability.

Follow-up Interval

An adequate follow-up period should tell us the adult outcomes of early school-age children with specific learning disabilities. Thus, a well-designed study should begin when a child enters elementary school and extend at least until the child reaches young adulthood. Studies that start with children at a later age may be studying biased samples (i.e., unremitting cases). Studies terminating before adulthood may provide limited information on ultimate adjustment, including marital, occupational, cognitive, and psychological status.

Sample Size

There is no magic number of subjects necessary for meaningful study. Nonetheless, a large sample does protect against some of the sampling artifacts inherent in small samples. A large sample, if representative of the population of disabled readers, increases the power to detect valid outcome effects.

Method of Sample Selection

The sampling procedure by which subjects are selected determines the generality of results from a study. The ideal sample is an epidemiological population survey. The next best is a sample drawn from an entire school district and the least desirable is a sample taken from a clinic, since this sample will be biased by the nature and referral base of the clinic.

Comparison Group

An adequate control group is a necessary yardstick for comparison. Only by knowing the relative outcomes of learning disabled children, as measured against those of non-disabled children, can one make appropriate statements regarding prognosis. Without a control group, one is unable to determine whether a good or poor outcome is specific to the index group.

Valid Reading Learning Measures

Clear-cut definitional criteria for classifying a child as learning disabled are necessary for interpreting results. Vague criteria make it impossible to determine the nature of samples, and thereby to interpret the meaning and generality of results. Without operational criteria for subject selection, one is unable to determine whether the index group was really learning disabled at baseline. In such a case, a good outcome would be potentially misleading and spurious.

As noted above, conclusions drawn from the box-score methods are themselves limited because important details of the studies are omitted. Methodologically weak studies may receive more weight than they deserve. Also, the box-score method treats results in terms of general criteria, without specifying the specific educational, occupational, psychosocial, and cognitive outcome variables. As such, it is unclear whether learning disabilities lead to school dropout, delinquency, or psychiatric problems. Furthermore, even modified boxscores do not give full indications of the methodological merit of individual studies. To evaluate the outcome results separately for each of the methodological criteria could lead to misleading conclusions if there were significant variability within studies on each of the criteria (e.g., an adequate follow up, but no control group or objective reading measures). Closer inspection of the better designed studies is necessary to make more definitive statements about the prognosis of learning disabled children.

Unfortunately, in the Schonhaut and Satz (1983) review, which spanned approximately 20 years (1959–1978), each study was found to be flawed on at least one of the methodological criteria mentioned above. Studies also varied considerably in overall quality of design. Thus, there was no definitive study to which one could turn for answers. In order to correct, in part, for these problems, a crude scale was developed, based on the preceding five criteria, permitting an evaluation of the aggregate methodological merits of each study. The criteria and scoring procedures are described in table II. While this scale is admittedly crude, it provided an objective procedure for ranking and classifying studies based on overall methodological merit.

Table II. Scale of Criteria for Rating Follow-up Studies

Criteria		Score
I.	Length of follow-up period	
	A. Follow up from before age 8 to after age 30	3
	B. Follow up period at least 10 years	2
	C. Follow up period at least 5 years	1
	D. Follow up period less than 5 years	0
II.	Size of sampling	
	A. At least 100 subjects	2
	B. At least 50 subjects	1
	C. Fewer than 50 subjects	0
III.	Adequacy of sampling procedures	
	A. Epidemiological population survey	3
	B. Entire school district	2
	C. Sample drawn from an entire school class	1
	D. Clinic sample	0
IV.	Adequacy of control	
	A. Matched control group of average readers	2
	B. Some control group or means of comparison	1
	C. No control group	0
V.	Adequacy of criteria for defining learning disabilities	
	A. Objective well-defined criteria	2
	B. Some attempt at systematic definitional criteria	1
	C. No attempt at systematic definitional criteria (e.g., vague criteria, diagnosis according to referral problem)	0

Table III shows the methodological ratings and outcomes for each study. A composite score of ≥ 6 was used to identify the methodologically stronger studies. Five of the 21 studies were classified as stronger (Rawson 1968; Howden 1967; Spreen 1978; Rutter et al., 1976; and Satz et al. 1978). The box-scores for these five studies was one good outcome and four poor ones. If one compares these box-score outcomes with the remaining 16 studies, table IV shows that unfavorable outcomes prevailed, regardless of methodological merit. However, an interaction was apparent between outcome and study merit. Three of the four good outcomes involved weaker studies, and four of the five stronger studies revealed poor outcomes.

Table III. Methodological Rating of Studies and Outcome

Study	I	II	III	IV	V	Composite Total	Outcome
1. Herman (1959)	3	0	0	0	0	3	P
2. Robinson and Smith (1962)	2	0	0	0	0	2	G
3. Carter (1964)	2	0	0	0	0	2	P
4. Silver and Hagin (1964)	2	0	0	1	0	3	M
5. Balow and Bloomquist (1965)	2	0	0	0	1	3	G
6. Howden (1967)	2	1	2	2	1	8	P
7. Preston and Yarrington (1967)	1	1	0	1	1	4	G
8. Hardy (1968)	1	0	0	0	0	1	P
9. Rawson (1968)	3	1	2	2	1	9	G
10. Bell et al. (1972)	0	1	1	1	1	4	M
11. Dykman, Peters, and Ackerman (1973)	0	1	1	2	0	4	P
12. Muehl and Forell (1973)	1	0	0	0	0	1	P
13. Gottesman, Belmont, and Kaminer (1975)	0	1	0	0	0	1	P
14. Kline and Kline (1975)	0	2	0	1	2	5	M
15. Rutter, Tizard, Yule, Graham, and Whitmore (1976)	1	2	2	2	2	9	P
16. Trites and Fiedorowiez (1976)	0	0	0	0	1	1	P
17. Rourke and Orr (1977)	0	0	1	2	2	5	P
18. Ackerman, Dykman, and Peters (1977)	0	0	1	2	2	5	P
19. Frauenheim (1978)	0	1	1	1	1	4	M
20. Satz, Taylor, Friel, and Fletcher (1978)	0	2	2	2	2	8	P
21. Spreen (1978)	2	2	0	2	0	6	P

*I, length of follow-up period; II, size of sample; III, adequacy of sampling procedure; IV, adequacy of control; V, adequacy of criteria for learning disabilities. Outcome = good (G), poor (P), mixed (M)

Table IV.   Outcome by Methodological Merit

Studies	Outcome Good	Mixed	Poor	Total
Strong[a]	1	0	4	5
Weak	3	3	10	16
Total	4	3	14	21

[a]Composite score ≥6.

The purpose of the present chapter is to provide a more updated review of the recent literature on the prognosis for LD children, using the preceding rating procedures to evaluate each study for methodological merit. These procedures will then be used to identify only the methodologically stronger studies which in turn will be combined with those from the earlier Schonhaut and Satz (1983) review.

CURRENT REVIEW

We were able to identify 12 additional studies that have been published since the Schonhaut and Satz (1983) review which included studies from 1959 (Herman) to 1978 (Spreen). One of the studies had multiple follow-up assessments (Spreen 1986; 1989a and b) and will be critiqued below. One other study (Bruck 1985) reported more recent data that were also presented in an earlier report (Bruck 1981). The current review includes studies from 1981 (Bruck) to 1993 (McKinney, Osborne, and Schulte). The general outcome results can be seen in table V. Without weighing scientific merit, they revealed three good outcomes, eight poor, and one mixed outcome. These box-score outcomes once again tend to show a preponderance of unfavorable outcomes.

Table V.   LD Outcomes: Recent Studies (*n* =12)

Good	Mixed	Poor
Finucci et al. (1985)	Levin et al. (1985)	Jaklewicz (1982)
Silver et al. (1985)		DeFries et al. (1983)
Bruck (1985)		Frauenheim et al. (1983)
		Zigmond et al. (1985)
		Michelsson et al. (1985)
		Spreen (1986, 1989a, b)
		Korhonen (1991)
		McKinney et al. (1993)

Box-Score Outcomes: 3(G), 1 (M), 8(P).

Each study was then rated in terms of the methodological criteria described by Schonhaut and Satz (1983). For purposes of brevity, only the methodologically stronger studies ($n = 7$) are listed as follows: (DeFries and Baker 1983; Finucci, Gottfredson, and Childs 1985; Bruck 1985; Zigmond and Thornton 1985; Spreen and Haaf 1986; Spreen 1989a and b; Korhonen 1991; and McKinney, Osborne, and Schulte 1993). Using these methodological criteria, one finds a much higher percentage of stronger studies in the recent literature ($7/12 = 58\%$) compared to the earlier review ($5/12 = 24\%$) [table III]. The box-score outcomes for these seven studies were two good and five poor. So, although the recent literature includes a higher number of methodologically stronger studies, unfavorable outcomes continue to prevail.

SUMMARY CRITIQUE OF STRONGER STUDIES

The following section provides a summary critique of each of the methodologically stronger studies in both the Schonhaut and Satz (1983) and current review. These combined studies (1959–1993) are presented in table VI by reported outcome and methodological rating. The box-score outcomes again point to unfavorable outcomes even with the methodologically stronger studies (three good, nine poor). It is interesting to note that none of the methodologically stronger studies revealed a mixed outcome. The following studies will be critiqued chronologically by outcome.

Table VI. LD Outcomes: Methodologically Stronger Studies (1959–1993) Schonhaut and Satz (1983) Criteria[a]

Good	Composite Score	Poor	Composite Score
Rawson (1968)	9	Howden (1967)	8
Finucci et al. (1985)	11	Ruttter et al. (1976)	9
Bruck (1985)	10	Satz et al. (1978)	8
		Spreen (1978)	6
		DeFries et al. (1983)	8
		Zigmond et al. (1985)	8
		Spreen (1986, 1989a, b)	8
		Korhonen (1991)	6
		McKinney et al. (1993)	7

Box-Score Outcomes: 3(G), 9(P).

[a]Merit Composite Score ≥ 6.

Good Outcomes

Rawson (1968) is one of the most widely quoted follow-up studies on learning disabilities. The 56 subjects in this study represented all the boys who attended the School in Rose Valley (Pennsylvania) for at least three years between 1930 and 1947. These subjects were rated by Rawson according to the Language-Learning Facility Scale, a largely subjective instrument developed by the author.

In 1964–1965, Rawson interviewed the subjects when they were 26 to 40 years old. She reported that 18 of the 20 dyslexic children had graduated from college and had had an average of six years of post-high-school education. This was slightly, but nonsignificantly, higher than the 5.45 years of post-high-school education obtained by the top 20 children on the Language-Learning Facility Scale.

The occupational achievement of Rawson's dyslexic subjects was also on a par with the average and above-average readers. The mean socioeconomic status (SES) of the dyslexics did not differ from the better readers; again, the difference was not significant. A majority of subjects in all of Rawson's groups fell into either SES Class I (professional or higher business) or Class II (subprofessional or middle business).

From these results, Rawson concluded that dyslexic children had a favorable prognosis. Several aspects of Rawson's study, however, restrict the generality of her findings. First, Rawson's sample consisted of extremely bright children from upper-class and upper-middle-class families. The Binet IQs of the children ranged from 94 to 185, with a mean of 130.8. No fewer than 46 of the children had fathers in SES Class I. Moreover, Rawson's criteria for classifying a child as "dyslexic" were unclearly specified. Therefore, it is not known whether some of these children would have been labeled "dyslexic" on more objective criteria. It is clear that Rawson's subjects are not representative of the average dyslexic child. While the study was based on an entire school population, that population was unlike the population of school children at large.

One may conclude from the Rawson study that intelligent, middle-class elementary-school children with some degree of reading difficulties may, with adequate opportunities, become productive adults. The study, however, is limited in its generality, and as such, does not tell us about the prognosis of less privileged dyslexic children. Nor does this seminal study report data on variables other than academic and occupational outcomes.

Bruck (1981, 1985) investigated the academic, occupational, social, and emotional status of 101 late adolescents and young adults who had been diagnosed learning disabled during childhood. This index group was contrasted with 50 non-learning disabled peers and 51 non-learning disabled siblings of the LD subjects matched for age, sex, and social class. The index group was followed until the ages of 17–29 years, representing approximately an 8–20 year follow-up period. Follow-up testing was given only to the index and peer control groups, although the parents and subjects of all these groups were interviewed. Testing was limited only to measures of reading, spelling, and math skills at follow up, although more extensive assessment data, including IQs, were available for the index group when they were referred to the McGill-Montreal Children's Hospital Learning Center for diagnosis and treatment many years earlier. The index group was selected from a list of 259 names of potential cases drawn from 5000 children referred to and diagnosed as LD in this center. From this list 156 families (60%) agreed to participate, from which 101 (39%) were recruited for testing. One should note that the index group represented approximately 2% of the original center population. The LD and controls came from middle- or higher-class backgrounds and included only 6% from lower working-class families. At entry to the center (Mean age = 8 years), IQ scores were in the average range (Mean = 103, SD = 11.22). All subjects had difficulties with written language, 75% were experiencing difficulties with math, and 45% were evidencing problems in visuo-spatial processing. Forty-three percent of the index group were performing in the severely disabled range (reading, spelling, and/or math), 31% were in the moderate range, and 27% in the mildly disabled range.

Although testing was limited to reading, spelling, and math skills at follow up, this study represented one of the few attempts to provide objective measures of achievement during late adolescence and young adulthood. Parental interviews were also conducted to obtain reports on psychosocial adjustment and educational attainment during this period. The results showed that many of the childhood problems in reading, spelling, and math persisted at follow up. However, despite this difficulties, most of the LD subjects had sufficient skills to further their schooling and occupational status. There were very few who remained non-readers or illiterate. Although the achievement and educational progress of the LD groups were consistently lower than peer groups, there were far fewer differences between the LD groups and their sibling controls. The reason for this outcome is that the peer group was selected by the LD subjects, who apparently identified more successful students as those whom they wished to be like. The peer group, unavoidably, became unrepresentative of the Canadian school population, thus necessitating sibling controls for many of the contrasts.

Bruck (1985) reported that a majority (59%) of the LD group had attended junior college or universities. The attendance record is somewhat inflated, however, because it included dropouts. By excluding dropouts, attendance rates in progress would lower to 42% (LD), 80% (Peer Control) and 50% (Sibling Control). Only 11% of the LD subjects had graduated from college (compared to 20% [peer] and 12% [sibling]).

Despite the relatively lower educational attainment of the LD subjects, they managed to obtain similar occupational status as compared to their sibling controls. Bruck (1985) also found no increased rate of school dropout, delinquency, alcohol, or drug abuse in the LD group, even when compared to the peer controls.

This study relied on parental reports of psychosocial adjustment at follow-up. Parents reported that their LD offspring had more problems in psychological adjustment than their peer controls. Results also showed that females experienced more social and emotional problems that tended to persist after childhood than did sibling or peer controls. This gender finding, also observed in the Spreen (1989 b) follow up, was explained in terms of culture sex-role stereotypes and expectations for female academic achievement. Consequently, violations of this stereotype were felt to impact more seriously over time on learning disabled females.

The Bruck study also found that childhood IQ and family SES were the best predictors of educational outcomes. Bruck stated that". . . these associations were strongest for those subjects at the extremes of each scale. For example, all subjects from lower-class backgrounds either dropped out of high school or did not continue their education beyond high school. Subjects who were successful in college programs had the highest childhood IQs" (p. 257).

Although the overall results of this landmark study were generally favorable in terms of academic and occupational adjustment, it should be noted that learning problems persisted in a majority of the LD subjects and that academic matriculation was slower and more difficult for many of those who attended junior colleges and universities. Although it was suggested that generally favorable outcomes were associated in part with early identification and remediation, it should also be noted that SES and IQ factors probably accounted for a major part of these good outcomes. Whether these effects were independent or group assignment (LD, control) remains unclear because of the absence of multiple regression analyses. Also, the reliance on interview data for psychological functioning at follow up weakens any firm conclusions that could be drawn on this important outcome domain. The interviews, largely subjective and subject to response bias, included no structured formats that would have permitted DSM-III-R Axis I or II diagnoses.

Finucci, Gottfredson, and Childs (1985) conducted a long, though variable, follow up (1–38 years) of two groups of subjects, one whose subjects had attended a private school for dyslexics (Gow School) and a control group of non-dyslexic subjects who had attended another private school (Gilman). Extensive test data (IQ and achievement) were available at school entry for the Gow students. At follow-up, only questionnaire data were available (education, occupation, marital status, family history, reading disorder, handedness) for 472/965 (49%) of the men who attended Gow (years 1940 and 1977) and for 384/753 (51%) of the Gilman alumni. Demographic data were available on a higher number of subjects in both groups, depending on the variable. The SES levels for both groups were generally high and consistent with subjects enrolled in independent college preparatory schools. The mean IQ (Stanford-Binet) was 117.9 for the Gow students, although their achievement quotients all fell in the severe disability ranges. No baseline IQ or achievement data were reported at school entry for the Gilman subjects.

The long-term academic and occupational outcomes were generally good for both groups, although the prevalence of college degrees was almost twice as high for the Gilman students (95% vs. 50%). Interestingly, the Gow students tended to interrupt their schooling more often than their controls (Gilman) and approximately three times as many Gow students took at least five years to earn a bachelor's degree. There was also a difference in types of degrees earned, with the majority of Gow students majoring in business and later matriculating into managerial work. In contrast, a majority of the Gilman students earned degrees in science and liberal arts with many matriculating into law, medicine, and science. Although many of the Gow subjects did not do so well as the Gilman subjects, and reported less interest and skill in reading and spelling, their attainments were nevertheless impressive given the severity of their childhood reading problems. The results showed that the educational and occupational outcomes of the Gow students was predicted by the initial severity of their reading, spelling, or arithmetic difficulties as well as by their responses to treatment (remediation) while in school. Greater initial severity in reading skill resulted in poorer long-term outcome (dose response), whereas successful responses to remediation resulted in more favorable outcomes. Family support was also shown to be predictive of good outcome in the Gow students.

This landmark study, while lacking in objective measures of reading, cognitive, and psychological function at follow up, nevertheless provides important data on long-term educational and occupational outcomes in bright subjects from more advantaged SES families.

Poor Outcomes

Howden (1967) followed 53 children who attended fifth- or sixth-grade classes in Springfield, Oregon, in 1942. The sample consisted of 22 "poor" readers, 22 "average" readers, and 9 "superior" readers. Classification into these categories was based on the relative reading performance of the students. Subjects more than 1 *SD* below the class mean were classified as poor readers, and those falling into the middle were considered average readers. Subjects were followed for an average of 19 years to when they were 29 to 35 years old. Follow-up assessment consisted of an interview and the Gates Reading Survey.

Results showed that the poor readers did not do so well on the Gates Reading Survey as the average and superior readers did. Poor readers also received fewer years of formal schooling and were more likely to have dropped out prior to graduating from high school. Likewise, the occupational status of the poor readers was below that of the average and superior readers. Howden's results apparently argue for a poor prognosis for reading-disabled children. There are, however, some reservations concerning this conclusion. For one, the SES of Howden's poor readers as children was lower than that of average and superior readers. This is a serious confound. If high SES predicts good outcome (Rawson 1968), then low SES may predict bad outcome, independent of childhood reading ability. What may be concluded, then, from this study is that children of lower SES who are also poor readers will tend to have poorer outcomes than higher SES students who are better readers—which does not say very much. Also, the outcome variable was restricted to measures of reading achievement at baseline and follow up.

The longitudinal project by Spreen (1978) provides the most extensive follow-up data gathered to date. Subjects in this study were 203 learning disabled children who were referred to the University of Victoria (British Columbia) Neuropsychology Clinic and the Nanaimo School District Educational Clinic. The mean age of these children, when they were first seen, was 9 and the average length of the follow-up period was 10 years. This follow-up investigation represented Phase 1 of the Victoria study. At baseline (Age range 8–12 years), subjects had to meet the following criteria: Verbal or Performance IQ > 69, no acquired brain damage during childhood, and no evidence of primary emotional disorders. Phase 2, which was conducted when the subjects were approximately 25 years old, will be critiqued later in this review (Spreen 1986; 1989 a, b).

Spreen divided the learning-disabled children into three groups, depending on the presence and severity of neurological signs. These exams were conducted by two experienced neurologists independent of and prior to the psychological assessments. The first group (IQ = 88) included children with at least one neurological "hard sign" or at least three "soft signs"; the second group (IQ = 95) comprised children with one or two neurological "soft signs"; the third group (IQ = 102) consisted of children with no neurological signs. The three groups of learning disabled children were compared with a control group of 52 normal achievers (IQ = 110), who were randomly selected by teachers. Socioeconomic status (SES) ranged primarily from lower middle to middle class in the LD groups. Structured interviews were conducted with both the subjects and their parents. Additional information was gathered from the Permanent (School) Report Card, a behavioral rating scale filled out by parents, the Bell Personal Adjustment Inventory, and ratings of subjects' interview behavior.

Results showed that in most aspects of educational, occupational, social, and psychological adjustment the outcomes of learning disabled children were worse than that of the control group. Sixty-two percent of the LD subjects dropped out of high school, only 12% entered college, and 46% were unemployed. According to Spreen (1988), their occupational levels were much poorer than that of the control group. Further analyses revealed that all LD subgroups had poorer emotional adjustment and social behavior than control subjects. Also, female subjects were found to have more social and emotional problems than the male LD subjects.

The major limitations of the study are that it used a clinic sample, and that it lacked strict criteria for classifying children as "learning disabled" at baseline. Because of this, the external validity of Spreen's findings is somewhat limited. Since the composition of the sample is unclear, it is difficult to generalize its findings to learning disabled children at large. Despite these limitations, the study is valuable because it provides information on many areas of social adjustment lacking in most other follow-up studies. In addition, it suggests that the presence and degree of neurological signs in learning disabled children may be important factors relating to prognosis. Finally, attrition was shown to be only 18% at the first follow-up (Ages 18–19).

Rutter et al. (1976) conducted a survey of children 9–10 years old who lived on the Isle of Wight in 1964–1965. These subjects were classified as "reading-backward," "specifically reading-retarded," or "normal" readers. Children were considered "reading backward" if they were at least 28 months below age-level reading, while they were labeled "reading retarded" only if they were 28 months below their expected age level and mental level (based on IQ). There was considerable overlap between the two reading-disabled groups, with 76 of the 86 reading-retarded children also counted among the 155 reading-backward children. The control group of 184 normal 9- to 10-year-old readers was a random sample selected from the remainder of the Isle of Wight population.

These children were followed five years to ages 14 or 15. Follow-up measures included a short form of the Wechsler Intelligence Scale for Children (WISC), the Neale Analysis of Reading Ability, the Schonell Spelling Test, and the Vernon Arithmetic-Mathematics Test. It was found that 56% of the backwardness group and 58% of the retarded group were more than 2 *SD*s below the mean in reading achievement. Also, only 4% of the backward readers and 2.5% of the retarded readers were at or above the age-level mean. The mean reading level for the combined group of disabled readers was that of the average 9-year-old, and spelling scores were even worse. Mathematics achievement of the disabled readers was also significantly below that of controls, although it was somewhat higher than the reading and spelling levels of these subjects. Compared to the reading-backward group, children with specific reading retardation showed (from ages 9–10 to 14–15) less improvement in spelling and reading, but more improvement in mathematics.

The Rutter et al. (1976) study appears to provide solid evidence that a majority of children who are severely disabled readers in middle childhood will continue to be disabled readers in adolescence. (Indeed, the disabled readers fell, over the course of the follow-up period, even further behind grade-level reading than at the outset of the study.) This study also provides evidence that reading disability may not represent an isolated deficit and may be associated with deficits in related academic areas, such as spelling and math. Similar observations have been reported in the Florida Longitudinal Project (Satz and Morris 1981; Satz et al. 1978) as well as the Bruck (1985) study. The differences at follow up in the Rutter et al. study between the reading-backward and the reading-retarded subjects indicate that subtyping of learning disabled subjects may provide useful prognostic information (i.e., the outlook for all learning disabled children may not be the same). In summary, it may be concluded from this study that the academic prognosis for many severely disabled readers aged 9 or 10 is poor.

The major weakness of the Rutter et al. study is the restricted length of the follow-up period. Children with learning disabilities who are younger than 9 or 10 may have a better prognosis. Also, adult prognosis for disabled readers may be better than the adolescent, as academic status would indicate. While it is reasonable to speculate that 14-year-old children reading at a 9-year-old level may tend to avoid college or drop out of school, it is still speculation. Moreover, with regard to the adult occupational, emotional, and social adjustment of these children, even less can be said. Despite these limitations, the Rutter et al. study provides valuable data on the prognosis of learning disabled children.

Satz et al. (1978) conducted a longitudinal study on the entire population of white male students entering kindergarten in Alachua County (Florida) public schools in 1970. Satz et al. obtained objective measures of subsequent second-grade classroom reading achievement and, based on these measures, classified subjects as "severely retarded" readers, "mildly retarded" readers, "average" readers, or "superior" readers. Out of a total of 426 students, 49 were considered severely retarded, 62 mildly retarded, 252 average, and 63 superior readers.

A follow-up study of these children was conducted three years later at the end of fifth grade. Again, objective measures of classroom reading were obtained, and children were classified as severely retarded, mildly retarded, average, or superior readers. Of the 49 children classified as severely retarded readers at the end of second grade, only 6% were average or above-average readers at the end of fifth grade. Also, only 17.7% of the mildly retarded readers were average or above in the fifth grade. Meanwhile, 30% of the average second-grade readers were mildly or severely disabled readers by the end of fifth grade. Only 3% of the superior second-grade readers were reading disabled in fifth grade. Similar findings were also reported using Wide-Range Achievement Test (WRAT) reading level scores as criteria; children who did poorly on the WRAT in second grade continued to do poorly in fifth grade. The subgroup of average second grade readers who became mild to severely disabled readers by the end of fifth grade represents a delayed onset group that has seldom been reported in the literature to date. This subgroup also warrants closer study in future prospective studies.

Results of the Satz et al. study suggest a grim prognosis for children having reading problems as early as second grade; very few children who had difficulty reading in second grade reached grade level by fifth grade. In contrast, several children who were average readers in second grade developed reading problems by fifth grade.

The major limitation of the Satz et al. study is the short follow-up period and the restricted focus on reading outcome. However, in conjunction with the Rutter et al. results, the Satz et al. study suggests that children who encounter reading problems in second grade may often have serious academic problems, encompassing reading, spelling, and mathematics, as adolescents.

DeFries and Baker (1983) reported a five-year longitudinal follow-up investigation of 125 reading disabled and 125 control children from grades 1 through 6. The probands and their affected siblings were part of the Colorado Family Reading Study which represented one of the most extensive family studies of reading disability reported in the 1980s. Subjects in both groups were ascertained by referral from personnel of local school districts and included subjects with IQs >90, no known emotional or neurological problems, and ages between 7.5 and 12 years. Control children were matched to probands on age, sex, grade in school, and home neighborhood. Families were typically English speaking, middle-class Caucasians. At the five-year follow up, psychometric data were available on 69 pairs of reading disabled and control children where the gender ratio was 5:1 males. Attrition was relatively high at follow up (45%). Although the Colorado Family Reading Study employed an extensive battery of psychometric tests, this study used only the PIAT (Reading Recognition, Comprehension, and Spelling) and two measures of psychomotor speed and processing (WISC Coding and Colorado Perceptual Speed) at baseline and follow up.

The results showed a significant improvement in all measures over time. While the rate of improvement in reading performance was similar in both groups, the slopes were parallel and reflected a similar gap or deficit between groups at both grades (1 and 6). In contrast, a significant group-by-time multivariate interaction was observed for the WISC coding task which revealed a different and slower rate of developmental change for the reading disabled group on this symbol processing task. Although this study lends support to those studies in this section showing persistence of the reading problem over time, the fact remains that both groups showed a similar rate of improvement. However, the group-by-time interaction for the symbol processing task suggests that despite this overall improvement in reading, the dyslexic group was falling further behind in information processing ability. This latter finding illustrates a need to examine other cognitive functions that may underline or mediate reading proficiency and outcome. It is instructive to note that the persistence of reading problems in this group between grades one and six is quite compatible with that reported in the Florida Longitudinal Project (Satz et al. 1978) for children between grades two and five and by Rutter et al. (1976) for children between the ages of 9 and 14. Although the Colorado Family Reading Project has published other data on genetic and neuropsychological factors in dyslexia, this study had more limited and focused

objectives which excluded relevant information on academic matriculation, grade retention, school dropout, employment, and psychological adjustment.

Zigmond and Thornton (1985) conducted a six-year follow-up
study of 105 LD children and a random sample of 118 non-LD children at grade 9 from a large, northeastern, urban school district. The
LD subjects who were identified relatively late in their schooling,
were part of an LD program. At baseline the LD group was shown to
be predominantly white (62%) and male (4:1). IQ (Otis-Lennon) and
Basic Skills Assessment (BSA) data were also available on both groups
as follows: LD (IQ = 80) versus NLD (IQ = 94.2), p <.001; LD (BSA
Read = 123.4) versus NLD (156.3), p <.001; LD (BSA Math = 125.0)
versus NLD (151.9), p <.001.

At the six-year follow up, school record and interview consent
forms were available for 60/105 LD and 61/118 NLD subjects who
were able to be located. However, IQ (WISC-R) and BSA consent
forms were available for only 35/61 LD and 38/61 NLD subjects.
Results showed approximately the same low IQ and BSA standard
scores for the LD group at both assessments. With respect to dropout
rates, the LD group showed a higher rate (54.2% vs. 32.8%). Grade
repetition was also higher in the LD group (35% vs. 16%), but it had
an equally ominous effect for both groups. According to the authors,
". . . Every NLD student who repeated a high school grade left school
before graduation: 90% of the LD students who repeated a grade
failed to graduate from high school" (p. 53). The final objective in this
study was to investigate employment status at follow up. Interestingly, employment status (employed and non-employed) was clearly
tied to dropout status, and not group assignment (LD vs. NLD). Those
subjects who managed to graduate were more likely to be employed
at follow up, despite group assessment. Unfortunately, grade matriculation and graduation were not associated with improved reading,
math, or IQ scores for the LD subjects. In fact, their scores were lower
than the NLD graduates and NLD drop-outs. In contrast to the good
outcome studies (Rawson 1968; Bruck 1985; Finucci, Gottfredson, and
Childs 1985), this study reported a bleaker outcome for grade retention, school dropout, IQ, and achievement skills for the LD group.
Unfortunately, no data were reported for SES level, but given the
urban setting, probably predominantly inner-city, a generally lower
SES background than that reported in the good outcome studies
above is suggested. Also, the low IQ levels for the LD group (Otis-
Lennon and WISC-R) would also be compatible with this impression.
The study results are also weakened by the small sample sizes, as well
as by the high consent refusals and attrition at the six-year follow up.

One might also argue that the late identification, and presumably minimal remediation efforts, coupled with low SES backgrounds, represented significant co-factors mediating outcome.

The Victoria Studies conducted by Spreen and colleagues followed the original cohort of 203 LD and 52 normal control children from childhood (Mean age = 9 years) to adolescence (Mean age = 18.9) [Phase 1] and to young adulthood (Mean age = 25 years) [Phase 2]. Three major studies have been reported on the Phase 1 and 2 follow ups (Spreen and Haaf 1986; Spreen 1989a, b) and are critiqued briefly below.

Spreen and Haaf (1986) used multivariate classification techniques (cluster analysis) to investigate cluster patterns at baseline (age 9) [Phase 1] and at follow up (age 25) [Phase 2]. The childhood clusters were based on two groups of LD subjects (n = 63 and n = 96) separately. The adult clusters were based on 124 LD and 46 controls. Cluster variables included the WRAT subtests and selected subtests from the WISC/WAIS. The results found similar subtypes at baseline for both groups as reported by other investigators. They comprised a visuo-spatial, linguistic, and articulo-graphomotor type. Of note, relatively few LD subjects emerged as having a specific reading or arithmetic deficit. While similar cluster patterns were observed at adulthood, the linguistic subtype was no longer present. This subgroup had a poorer outcome in terms of cognitive and academic performance, although the visuo-spatial subtype remained fairly stable across time. The results also showed that reading and arithmetic problems persist to adult age.

In a later study with some of this cohort, Spreen (1989a) investigated the stability of neurological soft and hard signs at baseline (age 9) and at adulthood (age 25) as well as their associations with different outcome variables (employment, monthly income, college or university attendance, and academic achievement). The neurological re-examination at age 25 was conducted independently by one of the two neurologists who was "blind" to the previous results. The results showed reasonable stability for many of the soft and hard signs, especially for those of relatively low frequency of occurrence (field defects, diplopia, dyspraxia). Interestingly, signs of uncoordination and graphaesthesia tended to disappear at age 25, whereas other signs such as synkinesis and intentional tremor actually increased with age. With respect to outcome, the frequency of neurological signs during childhood predicted poorer outcomes for grade completion, college attendance, monthly income, and employment.

The other Victoria study (Spreen 1989b) investigated the relationship between emotional disorders and neurological signs at ages

19 and 25 (Phase 1 and 2). Structured interviews and the Bell Adjustment Inventory were administered at age 18 years, whereas structured interviews and Minnesota Multiphasic Inventory (MMPI) were administered at age 25. Although sample size was not reported by LD groups and follow ups, attrition was reported to be 18% at Phase 1 and 19% at Phase 2. On parent ratings of being disorganized, emotionally dependent, and lacking appropriate social skills, a significant difference was found between LD subjects at age 18 with and without neurological signs. On the Bell Adjustment Inventory, elevated scores were found for problems at home, as well as social and emotional adjustment in all LD groups compared to the controls. Those LD subjects with hard neurological signs, however, differed from the other LD subjects on health adjustment. On the Bell Inventory a significant gender effect was found, showing that female LD subjects had elevated scores on emotional and social adjustment. This gender effect was also reported by Bruck (1985).

While many of the behavioral and emotional problems persisted in LD subjects at age 25, severity was attenuated, suggesting a less stressful time for many of these subjects after school-leaving age. Also, the gender effect disappeared.

At age 25, Spreen (1989a, b) also administered reading tests which revealed low scores for each of the LD subgroups (Grade levels = 7.3, 7.4 and 7.8 respectively) compared to the control group (Grade level = 10.3). Equally low scores were found for spelling and reading comprehension.

Despite some of the earlier concerns regarding subject ascertainment (school referrals to clinic), classification, and representation of the LD groups, which included children with probably congenital or acquired brain damage, the Victoria Project represents one of the landmark investigations on the long-term prognosis of LD children.

Korhonen (1991) investigated the stability and prognosis of neuropsychologically derived subgroups of LD children at grade three (ages 9–10) and at the end of grade six (ages 12–13). At baseline, 82 children with LD and 84 sex, age, and social-class matched controls were selected from the entire population of grade three children in Turku, Finland. Learning disabled children were identified by teachers from 27 schools, most of whom had taught the students for at least two years. Children were selected as having problems in reading, writing, spelling, or arithmetic. All children had a WISC-R Full Scale IQ of 80 or above. The severity of problems in the LD group was shown to be mild on a special reading and writing test; a vast majority of LD subjects were in regular classes at baseline and at follow up three years later. At follow up, 74 LD (80%) and 57 controls (68%)

were available for retesting on an extensive battery of neuropsychological tests. The paternal occupational status of both LD and control subjects was predominantly middle class. Interestingly, there was no change in WISC-R Verbal, Performance, or Full Scale IQ within LD or control groups over time, although the control group had an initial advantage in Full Scale IQ (109 vs. 98), but not at follow up. Four LD subtypes were found at both assessments (General Language, Visuomotor, General Deficiency, and Naming). These subtypes were then compared to reading and writing error scores on a non-standardized instrument developed by the authors. Results revealed a gradual improvement in reading and writing scores in all subtype groups, except for Naming. This latter finding is similar to that reported by Spreen and Haaf (1986) which also reported a poorer academic outcome in the language disorder subtype, but dissimilar to the Korhonen study which showed much improvement from grades 3 through 6. Although the LD group showed persistence of neuropsychological and reading difficulties at both baseline and follow up, approximately 36% of the LD children showed significant improvement in reading at follow up. This finding illustrates an important point—namely, that not all LD children fair poorly at follow up and may later have good outcomes in achievement. Unfortunately, the follow-up interval in this study was admittedly brief and limits any firm conclusions regarding recovery. It does relate, however, to the importance of identifying subgroups of LD children who later achieve good outcomes as well as non-disabled children who later achieve poor outcomes as in the Florida Longitudinal Project (Satz et al. 1978). While the follow-up intervals in both these studies were unfortunately brief, the results illustrate the importance of partitioning outcome variables into subgroups that eventually permit more focused tests to explain the different subgroups outcomes.

McKinney, Osborne, and Schulte (1993) investigated academic and LD outcomes in a small sample of 63 LD children identified in the first and second grades and retested five years later at the end of grade 6. A majority of subjects were African-American with lower SES status. This study also included a comparison group of 43 non-disabled controls. WISC-R and PIAT tests were administered to identify index and control children, all of whom had to have a Verbal or Performance IQ of 85 or above for inclusion. At follow up, 42 LD and 43 non-LD students were available for testing when they reached 11.5 years of age. The attrition rate of 33% was due to family mobility and/or non-consent responses. A major finding in this study, often unreported in other studies, was the lack of association between IQ and achievement discrepancy indices at grade one and achievement scores at follow up. However, results showed persistence of reading problems throughout grades 1 through 6. Although one third of the LD subjects were placed in mainstream classes at grade 5, their average overall achievement was still at the 30th percentile compared to the 49th percentile of the control subjects. For those LD subjects who still remained in special resource rooms, their overall achievement was even lower (20th percentile). The LD group also showed a grade retention rate of 64% by the end of grade 5. This was one of the few studies showing a decline in IQ and achievement in those LD subjects who also showed attention or behavior problems. Only two other studies in this review, both with stronger methodologies, reported similar declines over time (Rutter et al. 1976; DeFries and Baker 1983). This decline has previously been called the "Matthew effect" (Stanovich 1986). McKinney, Osborne, and Schulte (1993) interpreted this decline as follows:

> ". . . . Students with LD who are less task oriented complete less academic work and acquire less general knowledge, which exacerbates the learning difficulties associated with their primary disability. As a result, they are less able to profit from instructional opportunities and acquire less general and specific content-area knowledge. . . ." (p. 26)

This important study is weakened by the small and selected nature of the LD sample, the limited follow-up interval, and high attrition rate, as well as the higher prevalence of minorities with lower SES at follow up. The latter factors represent serious confounds with outcome. However, this study provides timely information on problems of case identification using a discrepancy index over time. The poorer outcomes for LD children with attention or behavior problems highlights the importance of co-morbidity factors on later outcome, particularly as it relates to the "Matthew effect."

CONCLUSIONS

The present review provides a summary critique of 12 of the methodologically stronger studies on the prognosis of leaning disabled (LD) children published between 1959 and 1993. These studies were selected from all known studies (33) published during this 34-year period directed toward the prognosis of LD children. Studies reporting the prognosis of ADHD children were excluded from this review. The 12 studies selected for critique were classified on the basis of criteria set forth in an earlier review by Schonhaut and Satz (1983).

Before discussing the general findings of these studies, it should be noted that the box-score outcomes for all studies, without regard to methodological strength, was predominantly unfavorable (Good = 7, Mixed = 4, Poor = 22), with only a minority showing favorable outcomes (7/33–21%). However, as pointed out in this review, such boxscores can be potentially misleading, especially if methodologically stronger studies were associated primarily with good outcomes. It was also felt that by restricting one's review to methodologically stronger studies, a clearer understanding of the prognosis for LD children over time would emerge. Unfortunately, this rationale, while probably a reasonable approach, was complicated by the fact that none of the stronger studies met all or most of the criteria for scientific merit.

Of all the criteria, length of follow up is one of the major determinants of long-term outcome. If sample size is small and attrition high, with no objective measure of outcome employed, or if so, restricted to a simple dependent variable (e.g., reading) one can see how the crucial follow-up interval could be weakened. If we consider only those studies employing a follow-up interval of 15 or more years, we find only five studies that meet minimal criteria for methodological strength (Howden 1967; Rawson, 1968; Finucci, Gottfredson, and Childs 1985; Bruck 1985; Spreen 1978, 1989a and b; and Spreen and Haaf 1986). Despite the relatively long follow up, these studies varied in terms of sample size, subject ascertainment, LD sample representation, and types of outcome assessed or reported (e.g., academic and/or psychosocial). Three of the studies reported good outcomes (Rawson 1968; Finucci, Gottfredson, and Childs 1985; Bruck 1985) and two reported poor outcomes (Howden 1967; Spreen et al. 1978–1989a and b). Unfortunately, two of these studies included very small sample sizes for the LD group (Howden 1967; Rawson 1968), who also differed in terms of IQ or SES. Howden's (1967) LD group (n = 22) which comprised lower SES subjects, had poor outcomes while Rawson's dyslexic subject (n = 20), who had high IQs (130) and high SES, had good outcomes. The importance of SES and/or IQ in predicting outcome was also seen in contrasting the Finucci, Gottfredson, and Childs (1985) with the Bruck (1985) and Spreen et al. studies (1978–1989 a, b). While educational matriculation was reported to be good in the Finucci and Bruck studies, differences still emerged between the LD and control subjects. Finucci, Gottfredson, and Childs (1985) showed that almost twice as many of the Gilman students (controls) graduated from college compared to the Gow students (95% vs. 50% respectively). However, the relatively high rates of academic matriculation in the Gow (LD) students, while substantially lower than the Gilman (control) students, were probably due to the high SES and IQs of these former preparatory school alumni. Mean baseline IQs for the

Gow students was 117. Note that Rawson's (1968) preparatory school LD students had a mean IQ of 130. By contrast, Bruck's (1985) LD subjects at baseline were apparently more severely impaired in reading, spelling, and math. They also comprised referrals to a clinic and had lower IQs (Mean = 103) and SES levels (approximately middle class). In this study, only 11% of the LD group graduated from college compared to peer controls (20%) and sibling controls (12%). The Bruck (1985) study showed that severity of childhood LD, lower IQ, and SES were the best predictors of poor outcome for educational attainment. Unfortunately, we do not know whether these co-factors were associated with parental reports of psychological adjustment problems in the LD females. The Victoria Project (Spreen 1978, 1989a and b; Spreen and Haaf 1986) provides the most dramatic contrast with the Finucci, Gottfredson, and Childs study (1985) in terms of IQ, SES, and neurological status on long-term outcome. The mean IQs of the three LD subgroups, which varied in terms of the presence or absence of neurological signs, were lower than the control group (IQ = 110) and ranged from 88–102. SES levels ranged primarily from lower middle to middle class. The LD group represented referrals from the school district and not private preparatory schools. As noted in other studies, the aggregation of lower IQ and SES, coupled with positive neurological signs, resulted in much poorer educational, occupational, and psychological adjustment at follow up. Sixty-two percent of the LD subjects dropped out of high school, only 12 % entered college, and 46% were unemployed at the 10-year follow up with little change at the 15-year follow up. Similar to the Bruck study (1985), psychological adjustment was poorer for the LD females. Unfortunately, in neither of these studies, which represent the only studies reporting a gender effect on long-term psychological adjustment, did the authors employ structured interviews for DSM-III-R Axis I and II disorders, or more comprehensive assessments of personality functioning. Even more surprising, no study to date in this review has yet examined family history of psychiatric disorder in index cases or controls.

For those studies which employed a much shorter follow-up interval, the results were essentially similar with respect to the importance of IQ and SES factors in predicting outcome. Also, in these studies, outcome variables primarily included data on grade completion, retention, and school dropout, as well as college attendance and/or graduation. Satz et al. (1978) followed a total school population of white boys from grade K to the end of grade five, while DeFries and Baker (1983) and McKinney, Osborne, and Schulte (1993) followed a sample of LD children and controls from grade one to grade six. Korhonen (1991) studied a sample of LD and control children from grade three to the end of grade six, and Rutter et al. (1976) followed two samples of LD children and controls from grade three to the end of grade nine. Finally, Zigmond and Thornton (1985l) followed a sample of late-identified LD children at grade nine for approximately five to six years. What is noteworthy in each of these studies is the relative persistence of reading and academic problems for many of the LD children during elementary, middle, and high school. As noted above, these findings were observed in even some of the longer follow-up studies, including a small, though unknown subgroup in the Finucci, Gottfredson, and Childs (1985) and Bruck (1985) studies, which reported generally good outcomes. The latter studies indicate that while a number of former LD subjects were attending or had graduated from college, not all were matriculating. Rutter et al. (1976) showed that while a majority of the LD subjects were showing persistence in reading, spelling, or mathematics at follow up, approximately 40% of the LD children had improved over the six-year period. Also, Korhonen (1991) showed that approximately 36% of the LD children in this study had improved significantly between grades three and six. It should be noted, however, that the LD sample was only mildly delayed in reading at baseline and almost all were in regular classes at baseline and follow up. Also, McKinney, Osborne, and Schulte (1993) showed that approximately 33% of his LD sample had been mainstreamed from special education classes by grade five, although their achievement test scores were still below their respective controls (30 vs. 49 percentiles, respectively).

These findings suggest that while childhood reading or learning problems may persist generally over time, the severity of the problems may decrease for some children who may also continue to pursue further schooling and occupational advancement. Whether these latter children also experience fewer psychological problems as adults still remains unknown. Nor do we know whether these adult changes in outcome are associated with a milder severity during childhood, or whether they are predicted by the protective effects of IQ, SES, and strong family support systems. Although the present review suggests the latter protective factors may predict better outcomes for some LD children, this hypothesis remains to be tested more definitively in future prospective studies. While the present review notes different trajectories for LD children, some of whom remain learning disabled over time, and some of whom acquire increasing academic skills and progress, we still lack clear understanding of those factors that predict these different trajectories. Nor do we know whether some children, during childhood, have a more delayed onset of reading or learning problems. Only data from Florida Longitudinal Project (Satz et al.

1978) comes to bear on this question. This prospective natural history study showed a subgroup of non-LD or average readers at the end of grade two who, at the end of grade five, became reading disabled. All other groups (LD and superior readers) remained essentially in the same outcome groups at the end of grade five. Jansky (1979) referred to this subgroup as "marginally ready," who, as the curriculum increased in complexity by grade four, were unable to compete with their peer controls and became learning disabled.

To conclude this review, it should be clear that larger and more epidemiological based studies are needed to address many issues and questions in this review. Because of the enormous costs involved in launching such projects, and in addressing many of the methodological and conceptual issues in this review, investigators will have to consider using data sets already collected in earlier large-scale multidisciplinary and multi-center projects. The National Collaborative Perinatal Project (NCPP), which was launched in the late 1950s and funded by NINCDS, represents one potential cohort. The NCPP recruited some 55,000 birth children from 12 different university/medical settings who were followed annually until age seven. The present authors (Lewis Lipsett, PI) have recently been funded by NINCDS and The March of Dimes to follow prospectively all children from the Providence cohort of the NCPP (4,140 subjects) who, at age seven, met criteria for LD based on WISC and WRAT discrepancy scores and were matched with a control group of non-LD children. The cohort is now approximately 35 years of age with approximately 70% residing within a 20-mile radius of Providence, Rhode Island. The current project seeks to investigate many of the long-term outcome variables included and recommended in this review. It is particularly focused on some of the differential trajectories not in this review with special attention to family history of LD, ADHD, and psychiatric disorder, birth and early developmental factors, types of early intervention programs, family support systems, and current cognitive and psychosocial functioning. It is hoped that this project will help resolve many of the problems addressed in this review.

REFERENCES

Bell, A. E., and Aftanas, M. S. 1972. Some correlates of reading retardation. *Perceptual and Motor Skills* 35:659–67.

Bruck, M. 1985. The adult function of children with specific learning disabilities: A follow-up study. In *Advances in Applied Developmental Psychology*, ed. I. E. Sigel. Norwood, NJ: Ablex.

Bruck, M. 1987. The adult outcomes of children with learning disabilities. *Annals of Dyslexia* 37:252–63.

DeFries, J. C., and Baker, L. A. 1983. Colorado family reading study: Longitudinal analyses. *Annals of Dyslexia* 33:153–62.

Finucci, J. M., Gottfredson, L. S., and Childs, B. 1985. A follow-up study of dyslexic boys. *Annals of Dyslexia* 35:117–36.

Fletcher, J. M., Francis, D. J., Rourke, B. P., Shaywitz, S. E., and Shaywitz, B. A. 1992. The validity of discrepancy-based definitions of reading disabilities. *Journal of Learning Disabilities* 25:555–61.

Frauenheim, J. G. 1978. Academic achievement characteristics of adult males who were diagnosed as dyslexic in childhood. *Journal of Learning Disabilities* 11:476–83.

Herjanic, B. M., and Penick, E. C. 1972. Adult outcomes of disabled child readers. *Journal of Special Education* 6:397–410.

Hermann, K. 1959. *Reading Disability: A Medical Study of Word-Blindness and Related Handicaps*. Copenhagen, Denmark: Munksgaard.

Howden, M. E. 1967. A nineteen-year follow-up of good, average, and poor readers in the fifth and sixth grades. Unpublished doctoral dissertation, University of Oregon.

Hynd, G. W., Semrud-Clikeman, M., Lorys, A. R., Novey, E. S., and Eliopulos, D. 1990. Brain morphology in developmental dyslexia and attention deficit disorder/hyperactivity. *Archives of Neurology* 47:919–26.

Jansky, J. J. 1979. Specificity and parameters in defining dyslexia. *Bulletin of The Orton Society* 29:31–38.

Kavale, K. A. 1988. The long-term consequences of learning disabilities. In *Handbook of Special Education: Research and Practice*. Vol. 2, eds. M. C. Wang, M. C. Reynolds, and H. J. Walberg. Oxford, England:Pergamon Press, Inc.

Korhonen, T. T. 1991. Neuropsychological stability and prognosis of subgroups of children with learning disabilities. *Journal of Learning Disabilities* 24:48–57.

Larsen, J. P., Hoien, T., Lundberg, I., and Odengaard, H. 1990. MRI evaluation of the size and symmetry of the planum temporale in adolescents with developmental dyslexia. *Brain & Language* 39:289–301.

Larsen, J. P., Hoien, T., and Odegaard, H. 1992. Magnetic resonance imaging of the corpus callosum in developmental dyslexia. *Cognitive Neuropsychology* 9:123–34.

McKinney, J. D., Osborne, S. S., and Schulte, A. C. 1993. Academic consequences of learning disabilities: Longitudinal prediction of outcomes at 11 years of age. [Special Issue: Risk and resilience in individuals with learning disabilities: An international focus]. *Learning Disabilities Research & Practice* 8:19–27.

Norman, C. A., and Zigmond, N. 1980. Characteristics of children labeled and served as learning disabled in school systems affiliated with Child Service Demonstration Centers. *Journal of Learning Disabilities* 13:542–47.

Pennington, B. F., Lefly, D. L., Van Orden, G. C., Bookman, M. O., and Smith, S. D. 1987. Is phonology bypassed in normal or dyslexic development? *Annals of Dyslexia* 37:62–89.

Pennington, D. G., and Smith, S. D. 1988. Genetic influences on learning disabilities: An update. *Journal of Consulting & Clinical Psychology* 56:817–23.

Pennington, D. G. 1991. The genetics of dyslexia. In *Annual Progress in Child Psychiatry & Child Development*, eds. S. Chess and M. E. Herzig. New York: Brunner/Mazel.

Rawson, M. B. 1968. *Developmental Language Disability: Adult Accomplishments of Dyslexic Boys.* Baltimore, MD: Johns Hopkins University Press.

Rutter, M., Tizard, J., Yule, W., Graham, P., and Whitmore, K. 1976. Research report: Isle of Wight studies, 1964–1974. *Psychological Medicine* 6:313–32.

Satz, P., Taylor, H. G., Friel, J., and Fletcher, J. M. 1978. Some developmental and predictive precursors of reading disabilities: A six-year follow up. In *Dyslexia: A Critical Appraisal of Current Theory*, eds. A. L. Benton and D. Pearl. New York: Oxford University Press.

Satz, P., and Morris, R. 1981. Learning disability subtypes: A review. In *Neuropsychological and Cognitive Processes in Reading*, eds. F. Pirozzolo and J. Wittrock. New York: Academic Press.

Schonhaut, S., and Satz, P. 1983. Prognosis of the learning disabled child: A review of the follow-up studies. In *Developmental Neuropsychiatry*, ed. M. Rutter. New York: Guilford Press.

Shaywitz, B. A., Fletcher, J. M., and Shaywitz, S. E. 1995. Defining and classifying learning disabilities and attention-deficit/hyperactivity disorder. *Journal of Child Neurology* 10:132–38.

Spreen, O. 1978. Learning disabled children growing up. A final report to Canada Health and Welfare, Monograph, University of Victoria.

Spreen, O. 1988. Prognosis of learning disability. *Journal of Consulting and Clinical Psychology* 56:836–42.

Spreen, O., and Haaf, R. G. 1986. Empirically derived learning disability subtypes: A replication attempt and longitudinal patterns over 15 years. *Journal of Learning Disabilities* 19:170–80.

Spreen, O. 1989(a). Learning disability, neurology, and long-term outcome: Some implications for the individual and for society. *Journal of Clinical & Experimental Neuropsychology* 11: 389–408.

Spreen, O. 1989(b). The relationship between learning disability, emotional disorders, and neuropsychology: Some results and observations. [Eleventh European Conference of the International Neuropsychological Society, 1988]. *Journal of Clinical & Experimental Neuropsychology* 11:117–40.

Stanovich, K. E. 1986. Matthew effects in reading: Some consequences of individual differences in the acquisition of literacy. *Reading Research Quarterly* 21:360–406.

Watson, B. U., Watson, C., and Fredd, R. 1982. Follow-up studies of specific reading disability. *Journal of the American Academy of Child Psychiatry* 21:376–82.

Zigmond, N., and Thornton, H. 1985. Follow-up of postsecondary age learning disabled graduates and drop-outs. *Learning Disabilities Research* 1:50–55.

Chapter • 12

Reading Dyslexia

Pasquale Accardo, M.D.

A TALE OF TWO SCHOOLS

I would like to describe two high schools in inner city St. Louis, Missouri. One is a public school in a rough neighborhood where personal safety is perhaps the overriding concern for many of the students. The dropout rate is approximately 50%. For those students who do graduate, the average reading level is fourth grade. If we consider a fourth-grade reading level to be marginal for literacy, then of those students who entered this public high school approximately 25% achieved something close to functional literacy. (In fact, most clinicians would place the cutoff for literacy several grades higher.)

The other high school is a private parochial institution with the highest academic standards. The dropout rate is virtually non-existent with 100% of the students, many with academic scholarships, going on to mostly prestigious colleges. All the students here graduate fluent in speaking, reading, and writing English, have taken at least one classical language (Greek or Latin), one modern foreign language, such as Spanish, French, Italian, or German, and often one more language, such as Russian or Chinese. Many of these students will have completed sufficient college credit courses in mathematics, English, science, and social studies to enter college at a junior-year level. When they graduate from high school, most of them already have reading levels above those of the average college senior.

If a student were to be administered a reading achievement test and score at an age- and grade-appropriate level on such a test (say, a standard score of 100), he might very well function as an honor student in the first high school. That same student would never have been accepted into the second school or would have had to struggle to keep up with the work. That there are tremendous social and emotional differences between the student bodies of both schools is obvious. Although some of the differences are trivial, such as the private prep school's being all male and requiring uniforms; many are not. The two institutions were specifically selected as extreme examples of the significant extrinsic variables that most researchers are forced to ignore in their pursuit of something called pure dyslexia. Nevertheless, the impact of a specific problematic reading level cannot be wholly explained by or wholly explained away by such differences. Neither is it possible to ignore these differences by simplistic references to the latter school's ability to select the best and brightest students.

A student with a standard score of 100 in reading achievement may or may not, in fact, have a genuine reading problem. If one looks only at the reading score and ignores the total picture of a child's learning, academic, developmental, medical, and social history, there simply is no way to know. The isolation of reading researchers who confine their diagnostic assessment of reading problems to educational tests alone, raises serious questions as to the relevance of their findings in the real world. Their isolation undermines the validity of their own research. With an average reading achievement level, no student should experience serious difficulties in an average grade school or high school. Since college programs allow a large amount of self-selection in choosing both programs/majors and individual courses (as well as teachers), fewer students will be at first identified as reading disabled at the college level (unless their first difficulties occur with the need for SAT modifications). If, however, the bright student with only an average reading ability attempts to go on to professional schools of medicine or law, he often quickly finds that the rigid modes of teaching and testing, as well as the high pressure to cram in a tremendous volume of factual knowledge over a very short time period (i.e., to digest and regurgitate a very large amount of reading material), generates previously unsuspected learning difficulties. A standard score of 100 for reading represents a significant disability for students trying to negotiate such a professional school curriculum.

Medical schools have experienced a notable increase in students with learning disabilities over the past decade. Over the past five years, the incidence of learning disabled medical students went from 1.3 to 2.9 per school (Section for Student Programs 1994). Clinical experience suggests that the majority of these are reading disorders (Accardo et al. 1989), but the reported doubling probably still represents a significant underestimate. On the one hand, the rise of this "new problem" might suggest that the educational system has succeeded in preparing students with learning problems to compete more successfully at the professional school level. On the other hand, it would appear that most of these learning disabled students were missed earlier on and only became aware of their disability when confronted with "high output failure" of their self-discovered compensatory skills.

It seems needless to say that problems encountered with the more gifted and talented students are found at the opposite end of the IQ spectrum as well. Children with Down syndrome will typically score quite low for grade and for age on a test of reading achievement. Their scores identify them as needing help in reading, but this will have already been recognized by the school system as part of a more generalized need for academic support. This is not always the case with other mental retardation syndromes. The inner city clinic that I direct evaluated 1,000 children last year. Included in this number were three students at the junior high school and high school levels placed in regular education classes without any special help despite being referred by their parents because of generally low academic achievement and, specifically, poor reading skills. All these students tested in the mentally deficient range, not borderline, with IQs of 50 and below. The diagnosis of mental retardation was confirmed in each case by supplementing the psychometric test data with detailed developmental histories, as well as measures of adaptive skills and other relevant functional domains. None of these children had dyslexia or any other specific reading problem. Furthermore, two of the three had medical conditions causing or complicating their mental retardation that should have been recognized earlier. School-based multidisciplinary assessment teams should not consider developmental diagnoses final without an appropriate developmentally oriented medical evaluation (Accardo 1995).

IS DYSLEXIA MORE THAN A READING DISABILITY?

Dyslexia is a developmental disability that shares many general characteristics with its parent group of neurological disorders. All developmental disabilities are trait disorders in which an individual with the disability performs, in the affected area of higher cortical function, more like a normal, but younger child. The impaired functioning might be general cognitive ability (global intelligence in mental retardation); reading and mathematics (poor academics in a neurologically based specific learning disability); reading (low reading achievement scores in dyslexia); mathematics (low mathematics achievement scores in dyscalculia); written language (illegible handwriting in dysgraphia); language (poor speech and language in phonological disorders and developmental disorders of language); fine motor coordination (clumsiness in apraxia); and executive function (inattention, impulsivity, and hyperactivity in attention deficit hyperactivity disorder) (Accardo 1996).

None of these disability subgroups is homogeneous. In mental retardation, for example, there are literally hundreds of genetic, metabolic, and dysmorphic syndromes that account for less than half of the currently identified population with mental retardation. The majority of cases still remain with uncertain or unknown etiology. Different mental retardation syndromes can exhibit markedly diverse physical, neurological, cognitive, and neurobehavioral profiles as well as being associated with different organ systems. In the past, most such etiological conditions were thought to be exclusive for mental retardation. While this remains true for certain conditions such as Down syndrome, it now appears that some of the most common etiologies are not often associated with mental retardation. Fragile X syndrome and fetal alcohol syndrome are much more likely to be associated with learning disabilities, attention deficit hyperactivity disorder, and other emotional and neurobehavioral diagnoses. Whatever the estimated prevalence rate for dyslexia, one can expect that it, too, like other developmental disabilities, exhibits a continuum of severity.

In the real life clinical situation, isolated dependence on statistical cutoffs that may be appropriate for epidemiological studies (Shaywitz et al. 1992) can readily be seen to be inaccurate, if not dangerously misleading, when mechanically applied to individual cases. Incidence/prevalence statistics for dyslexia are more reflective of the epidemiological bias or bureaucratic ideology of the reporter than of anything in the real world. Using a percentile score derived from a group-administered achievement test to identify reading disability in a population; or utilizing an individually administered reading test in isolation to diagnose a child with a reading disorder violates common sense. An individual intelligence test presents more well-defined psychometric properties than either of the above screening approaches; yet its results are only supportive of mental retardation and insufficient to validate such a developmental diagnosis in the absence of other information. The more loosely structured reading tests that are generally available should be considered even less capable of supporting meaningful and definitive diagnostic classifications. Such an approach might appear to some as simple and even elegant as part of a research protocol, but it is never permissible in the clinical situation to diagnose a developmental disability, any developmental disability, on the basis of a single test score or even on the basis of multiple test scores independently of clinical judgment. Most state plans in conformity with federal regulations even require more than one discipline to assess a child before the diagnosis of a developmental disability can be affirmed.

Apart from the fact that the act of reading is complex and involves much more than "phonological awareness" (something that Huey was aware of as early as 1908), any individual example of difficulty in reading must occupy a specific point on a spectrum that goes from the extreme of outstanding readers to children with severe dyslexia. Along the way, certain classifications may be distinguished: adequate readers (persons who have no reading disability but whose preferred learning style is more visual than auditory); weak readers (students whose pattern of test scores suggests a learning disability in reading, but who do not achieve the defined research or school cut offs required for formal diagnosis despite the fact that they are struggling with reading, yet not failing); children with a definite diagnosis of reading disability; and cases of severe dyslexia (intelligent children who after years of intensive intervention will, nevertheless, grow up to be adults who cannot read). Although the term dyslexia suggests a specific condition and can be useful to attract both educational resources and research funding, reading disorders are really (but not simply) one subcategory of neurologically based specific learning disabilities.

This is not to say that there are not more specific subtypes of reading disability that might be considered "pure dyslexia" and from which a great deal might be learned of the psychological processes that underly reading. Such cases probably do exist. However, most of the current research on dyslexia effectively ignores the associated symptoms of more diffuse brain involvement by utilizing none or highly superficial screening procedures to identify their presence. The assessment process to diagnose or rule out a co-morbid presence of, say, an associated attention deficit disorder, cannot be achieved with a screening instrument such as a Connors questionnaire with its sensitivity of just over 60%. Yet, it is rare to find a paper on dyslexia that goes beyond such a simplistic measurement to declare their subject population free of associated disabilities. The evaluations for other neurocognitive and neurobehavioral conditions are typically no better. Confused thinking at the research level can only contribute to increased public confusion.

A recent poll (Roper Starch Worldwide 1995) confirms what might otherwise have been suspected. After a quarter of a century of the Education for All Handicapped Children (PL 94–142) and all its later amendments and reenactments and the establishment of a special education industry, both the teaching profession and the American public, as a whole, continue to demonstrate widespread misunderstanding and woeful ignorance of the nature and treatment of all forms of learning disability. Indeed, they remain skeptical as to the very existence of such conditions. The lay conception of dyslexia in an otherwise bright child who sees letters reversed on the page, along with a wealth of more scientific information, has had little impact on popular misconceptions. In the past two presidential elections, populist candidates have courted public approval with a platform to do away with all special education supports.

The sympathy generated by the highly emotional picture of a child of average intelligence who just needs a bit more help to learn how to read, simply is not there. The clear definition of learning disabilities as neurologically based developmental disabilities needs to be promulgated more widely. Dyslexia (specific reading retardation) in children needs to be sharply differentiated from the laudable but utterly distinct concerns of the campaign against (adult) illiteracy. Developmental learning disability needs to have objective diagnostic parameters defined (both inclusive and exclusive). Congressional rumors about the negative impact of "designer disabilities" (such as the potential inclusion of any child with bad behavior under the rubric of attention deficit hyperactivity disorder with eligibility for SSI payments, along with the fear that some parents might be training their children to misbehave in order to qualify for such benefits) on the federal budget, need to be answered with clinical science and not with social planning agendas.

One of the first steps the clinician undertakes in the parent counseling of a child newly diagnosed as learning disabled in reading is demystifying the diagnosis and its implications. Next is assessing etiology and levels of functioning accurately and assisting the family in lining up resources for effective intervention. Such a comprehensive approach to a child with dyslexia ought to be routinely available to families, but this is not always the case. All too often the reading problem is viewed and interpreted in confusing isolation as a "school problem." On a broader scale, public education must proceed at a more intense pace if funding to continue existing support services is to improve and even increase. Current research on the efficacy of diverse intervention strategies is not so positive as to present an easy sales pitch to a generally under-educated and misinformed voting public. While it is not appropriate to recommend a research moratorium, it does seem foolish to continue developing more intensive and more expensive treatments in a society unlikely to expend the resources to implement them. (Both medical and educational research here seem to share an identical constraint.) Public education needs to be the number one priority for everyone actively involved in the field of reading disorders.

FUTURE DIRECTIONS

The presentation on which this chapter is based was originally entitled "Future Directions" with the intent of predicting the future of the concept of dyslexia along with the clinical and research diagnosis and treatment of reading disabilities. Prophecy maintains a U-shaped curve in that it is easy to predict the immediate future and even easier to predict the distant future, but difficult to predict the future that lies between.

With regard to the immediate future, things change slowly. Educational and clinical practices tend to change by decades rather than by years. The research findings reported in the other chapters of the present volume are still essentially state of the art two years after their initial course presentation; their numbers may have grown larger, the correlations tighter, and the statistics a bit more polished; but startling new directions are unlikely. A book or conference on dyslexia five years from today will look and sound very similar to the present overview. This resemblance is not necessarily because we have uncovered all that there is to know about reading disorders, but more simply, because it reflects the correctness and inescapability of the bulk of those observations upon which all theories and therapies of dyslexia must be based.

The same could be said for all branches of science. In 1895, Morgan Robertson published a novel describing the sinking of an unsinkable luxury liner, in the Atlantic Ocean after collision with an iceberg. He wrote this a full dozen years before the *S.S. Titanic* transformed his accurately detailed fiction (heavily based on then current shipbuilding speculations) into prophecy (Pedler 1981). Similarly, in 1909 Homer Lea published a novel, *Valor of Ignorance,* and Hector Bywater brought out a fictional account of *The Great Pacific War: A History of the Japanese-*

American Campaign of 1931–1933 in 1925. These books described with such incredible prescience the Pacific war that would not actually take place until 1941–1945, that the writers were thought to have inspired large parts of the Japanese "War Plan Orange" (Bloom 1990). As experienced military observers, the two authors merely wrote out possible scenarios that took accurate account of current advances in military technology and the geopolitical terrain of the situation in the Pacific. What looked like prophecy was only the short term application of current military science. These examples are simply validations of Clarke's Third Law according to which any sufficiently advanced technology will appear as magic to the uninitiated.

Long term prophecy is even easier (Darwin 1952). A million years from now there will be no dyslexia or reading disorders. Advances in genetic manipulation, neuroscience interventions, and educational techniques will have eradicated the problem. Indeed, the problem should be insignificant by the fourth millennium, if not by the twenty-second century.

THE FUTURE OF READING

> Words and the meaning of words predispose the child to think and act automatically in certain ways. The alphabet and print technology fostered and encouraged a fragmentary process, a process of specialization and detachment. Electronic technology fosters and encourages unification and involvement. (McLuhan and Fiore 1967)

A separate but related question concerns the future of reading itself. One of the major reasons that the knowledge of dyslexia is barely a century old is that universal literacy has only recently been considered a desirable world-wide goal. A century ago there were many occupations that did not require literacy, and economic pressures drove many children into the workplace instead of the schoolroom. One could survive in that world without being able to read.

Over the past century, we have moved towards creating a society where literacy has become essential. Even menial lower-level service jobs have increasingly higher literacy requirements hidden in such things as the need to read want ads, to fill out job applications, to use various training and technical manuals, and to file tax forms. Paradoxically, with the peaking of this dramatic escalation in the need to read, teaching and media technology are advancing at an even more rapid pace to make reading obsolete. Page text is being replaced by books on tape and electronic data bases. It has even been suggested that a large part of the cultural wars to get certain titles included in the educational canon is due partly to the fact that students will, at most, read only those few books on the required list. They have preferred usually electronic sources for facts, learning, entertainment, and leisure.

It is a matter of great concern to many social observers that increasing computerization is having a negative impact on young children's reading skills. Elementary school students can still decode type, but they no longer think in terms of books. Electronic post-modernity is charged with contributing to a fragmented sense of time, short attention span, impatience with sustained inquiry, divorce from the past, a lessened sense of geographical space, a weakened faith in institutional structures, and the loss of any strong vision of the future (Birkerts 1994). As the clarity of language erodes, many unexpected and even deleterious effects may occur, many of which were already implicit in earlier revolutions in modern philosophy and post-modern literary theory. The electronic media have followed, rather than led the dramatic changes society is experiencing. Nevertheless, it is probably true that this radical electronic change is on the same order of magnitude as the history-making revolution heralded by Gutenberg's invention of moveable type.

What is often forgotten in the clinical management of a child with dyslexia is that reading is not an end in itself. One can observe certain children and adults with mental retardation or autism who have such phenomenal decoding skills that they can fluently "read" any text. But their comprehension of what they are reading is virtually nil. (This phenomenon is sometimes referred to as "hyperlexia.") The child or adult with dyslexia is often in the exact opposite situation: he cannot decode the written text into its phonological equivalent. If, however, that same written text is translated into the spoken word by some other technique such as an audiotape, a speaking computer, or another person reading out loud, his comprehension of what has been "read" can be exemplary.

Both clinicians and social critics need to understand the full implication of this postulate that reading is never an end in itself. Reading is merely a technology, a technique to store and transfer information. It is one technology among others, and now an eminently replaceable one. Two millenia ago, when the oral tradition gave way to the written text, philosophers predicted dire consequences to civilization. For thinkers such as Plato (Phaedrus 275 a–b), the introduction of the arts of reading and writing implied an end to civilization: "If men learn this [the alphabet], it will implant forgetfulness in their souls; they will cease to exercise memory because they rely on that which is written, calling things to remembrance no longer from within themselves, but by means of external marks. What you have discovered is a recipe not for memory, but for reminder. And it is no true wisdom that you offer your disciples, but only its semblance, for by telling them of many things without teaching them you will make them seem to know much, while for the most part they know nothing, and as men filled, not with wisdom, but with the conceit of wisdom, they will be a burden to their fellows" (R. Hackforth 1961). Before the advent of writing, epic poems and other culturally significant material were committed to memory. Homer's blindness emphasizes his independence of any written text.

Technology can inform thought patterns. Plato was correct in saying that using a new technology would have an impact on how people thought, but he had no reason to assume that because they thought differently, they would necessarily think less clearly. A large part of the concerns with the advent of print, the invention of moveable type, and the coming of the computer, centers on a strongly democratic and levelling tendency inherent in all these technologies. Someone so unintelligent as not to be able to read would now have the same access to information locked away in books as the best of readers.

Lest the above argument be taken to give spoken language precedence over the written word, let it be remembered that thought is not indissolubly linked to language (Weiskrantz 1988). With the appropriate social supports, people who are deaf (Groce 1985) and people who elect to use sign language (Barakat 1975) live intelligent and fulfilling lives.

There are aspects about acquiring information through print media that will not readily translate when the same information is acquired by other means. If reading becomes inessential, then those patterns of thinking and the social patterns that are affiliated with them will need to be identified and taught by other means.

REFERENCES

Accardo, P. 1995. The bridge not crossed. *Their World.* New York: National Center for Learning Disabilities.

Accardo, P. J. 1996. *The Invisible Disability: Understanding Learning Disabilities in the Context of Health and Education.* Washington, DC: The National Health and Education Consortium and Learning Disabilities Association of America.

Accardo, P. J., Haake, C., and Whitman, B.Y. 1989. The Learning disabled medical student. *Journal of Developmental and Behavioral Pediatrics* 10:253–58.

Barakat, R. 1975. *Cistercian Sign Language: A Study in Non-verbal Communication,* Cistercian Study Series, Number 11. Kalamazoo, MI: Cistercian Publications.

Birkerts, S. 1994. *The Gutenberg Elegies: The Fate of Reading in an Electronic Age.* Boston, MA: Faber and Faber.

Bloom, J. 1990 Predicting future wars, half a century ago. *Strategy and Tactics.* May/June, 134:22–6, 55–7.

Darwin, C. G. 1952. *The Next Million Years.* Garden City, New York: Doubleday.

Groce, N. E. 1985. *Everyone Here Spoke Sign Language: Hereditary Deafness on Martha's Vineyard.* Cambridge, MA: Harvard University Press.

Hackforth, R. (translator) 1961. Phaedrus In *The Collected Dialogues of Plato.* eds. E. Hamilton and H.Cairns. Princeton, NJ: Princeton University Press.

Huey, E. B. 1908. *The Psychology and Pedagogy of Reading* reprinted 1968. Cambridge, Massachusetts: MIT Press.

McLuhan, M., and Fiore, Q. 1967. *The Medium Is the Massage: An Inventory of Effects.* New York: Bantam Books.

Pedler, K. 1981. *Mind Over Matter.* London: Thames Methuen.

Roper Starch Worldwide. 1995. Learning Disabilities And The American Public: A Look At America's Awareness and Knowledge. Poll prepared for the Emily Hall Tremaine Foundation.

Section for Student Programs. 1994. Learning disorders in medical students: Survey of U.S. Medical Schools. Association of American Medical Colleges.

Shaywitz, S. E., Escobar, M. D., and Shaywitz, B. A., Fletcher, J. M., and Makuch, R. 1992. Evidence that dyslexia may represent the lower tail of a normal distribution of reading ability. *New England Journal of Medicine* 326:145–50.

Weiskrantz, L. (ed.) 1988. *Thought Without Language.* Oxford: Clarendon Press.

Index

WITHDRAWN